Common Diseases and Syndromes of Body Pain

The Compiled Rheumatic and Neuropathic Book Titles of Jim Lowrance

By: James M. Lowrance © 2012

SECTION ONE:

Peripheral Neuropathy Causes and Treatments

Conditions of Nerve Pain and Dysfunction

TABLE OF CONTENTS:

Common Diseases and Syndromes of Body Pain

INTRODUCTION:

Some estimates by medical research groups state that up to 20 million Americans suffer from some form of peripheral neuropathy (PN) and this number is much higher when worldwide statistics are considered. One major reason for the rise in incidence for these conditions of damage to the nerves in the body that results in pain and dysfunction in them is the increase in cases of diabetes and pre-diabetic syndromes. With the past few passing decades, an increase in consumption of simple carbohydrates (refined sugars and starchy foods), as opposed to complex carbohydrates (fruits, vegetables, nuts and grains) and the decrease in physical exercise, has contributed to an exponential increase in metabolic syndromes and later-life diabetes within the general population.

With bad diet practices and obesity starting at earlier ages In these modern times, than in decades-past, the term "adult onset" is not as often used in referring to later-life development of diabetes. This epidemic of endocrine disease affecting glucose regulation in the body that is most-often referred to as "Type II Diabetes", is now affecting large numbers of children and young people, at an alarming rate of increase.

Common Diseases and Syndromes of Body Pain

This has also greatly increased the number of people suffering symptoms of PN, with up to 70% of patients with diabetes suffering mild to severe nerve damage, due to chronic glucose dysregulation.

There are many other causes of PN however, including old age, viral infections, nutritional deficiencies, various autoimmune diseases, dysfunction of the arterial system (blood circulation) and drug-use of both prescribed types and varieties of illegal drugs and the use of alcohol for recreational purposes (i.e. to achieve a high or a state of sedation).

Within the chapters that follow, I will be addressing the types of symptoms involved in PN diseases, the types of nerves that can be affected and treatments that are administered to treat underlying causes of PN and to directly address its symptoms. It is my sincere hope that this book will serve to gain its readers, a good general education on the subject of Peripheral Neuropathy.

CHAPTER ONE

My Personal Battle with Peripheral Neuropathy (PN)

In the year 2003, I was diagnosed with autoimmune thyroid disease, my low-functioning thyroid (hypothyroidism) being caused by a condition common to the populations of industrialized countries, called "Hashimoto's thyroiditis" (also referred to as "chronic lymphocytic thyroiditis"). In my case, some of the more concerning symptoms that manifested with the disease, were rheumatic ones (joint and muscle pain) as well as general body aches that felt similar to what one might experience with a flu virus. I also experienced what I now can look back and recognize as the beginnings of PN symptoms.

I can remember periods of time that my hands and feet would tingle and my feet especially would experience mild burning sensations, especially at night after retiring to bed for a night's sleep. I also remember feeling occasional pains in my arms, that would radiate out to the ends of my fingers but these were less-frequent at the time, than were the general body aches.

These pain and sensory sensations as related to PN would be caused by problems involving "sensory nerves" (the ones that conduct senses of feel, including pain, body position and temperature).

My more concerning symptoms at the time and in the years that followed were muscle weakness and easy fatigue-ability that I noticed to be especially prominent in my arms and legs and that seemed to slowly progress, rather than to improve with my hypothyroid treatment. The treatment consisted of a daily dose of prescribed thyroid hormone replacement therapy. Muscle weakness when caused by PN, is a manifestation of problems with the "motor nerves" (the ones that help to control muscle movements and strength). It was my belief and that of two different doctors that I attended, that I likely had a co-morbid condition such as fibromyalgia and/or Chronic Fatigue Syndrome.

One of my doctors felt that it was possible that my symptoms were tied directly to my elevated thyroid antibodies levels (positive thyroid antibodies help to confirm the diagnosis of thyroid autoimmunity diseases). One of my antibody levels, called the "anti-thyroglobulin" (TG) was elevated at "537" with normal values being anything below 40. This meant mine were almost 500 points above normal.

Common Diseases and Syndromes of Body Pain

My "anti-thyroidperoxidase" antibodies (TPO) were also elevated but not as significantly. These were positive at "120" with normal values being anything below 35.

Due to my TG antibodies being significantly elevated, my thyroid-treating doctor at the time (now retired) placed me on a short-term corticosteroid steroid (prescription anti-inflammatory drug) to see if this might improve my rheumatic symptoms, including the muscle weakness and fatigue-ability. I did experience a short-lived improvement but the effects diminished shortly after I discontinued the steroid medication. After several more years of suffering these unrelieved symptoms and having two vitamin deficiencies found in my blood tests (Vitamin D and B12) I asked my MD for a referral to a neurologist, early in the year 2010.

The new doctor tested me for yet other vitamin deficiencies and I was found to be deficient in vitamin E as well and in-fact it was the most severe deficiency found via blood testing, at "0.4" with normal values being between 3.0 and 16.0. I have since been treated for these deficiencies and have experienced some improvement in the PN symptoms, especially the sensory ones involving pain sensations. My muscle weakness – the motor nerve ones have also improved to some degree but not significantly.

Common Diseases and Syndromes of Body Pain

I do however believe that I may see further improvement in coming months, my treatment as of now having only been administered for approximately 6 months at the time of this writing.

In addition to blood testing, my neurologist also administered Nerve Conduction Studies (NCS), which is testing that measures the "amplitudes" of large fiber nerves within the body (the efficiency of them in conducting electrical impulses). It was found via the results of this testing, that I had slightly below-normal and in some cases, low-normal amplitudes in several of my large fiber nerves.

I was also tested for small fiber neuropathy, via a test called "hole punch biopsy", which takes core tissue samples from the lower leg and analyzes them for damage in the small nerves. My results were within normal limits, however, the reviewing-physician noted that mine did show some evidence for the beginning of small fiber nerve damage.

Through extensive research, I found that PN is strongly associated with thyroid diseases, especially when treatment is delayed or the thyroid hormone imbalances caused by them becomes severe.

It would appear from medical research that has been published in recent years, that all endocrine diseases, meaning those affecting the hormone regulating glands in the body (i.e. the pancreas, thyroid and adrenal glands) all have potential to cause various degrees of PN. Thyroid patients with autoimmune hyperthyroidism (Graves' disease) for example, have been found to be especially vulnerable to PN symptoms and nerve damage from excessive thyroid hormone levels in the body and inflammation from auto-antibodies.

In regard to vitamin deficiencies and other nutritional imbalances; these may possibly be the most common cause of PN worldwide, with diabetes being the most common cause in the more industrialized countries, including the US. More about the relationship of PN to diabetes and nutritional deficiencies will be addressed in chapters that follow.

CHAPTER TWO

Nerve Damage from Diabetes and Metabolic Syndromes

Nearly 18 million Americans currently have a diagnosis of diabetes and over 1.5 million new cases are diagnosed yearly. It is believed by reputable medical research groups that up to 6 million Americans have diabetes but remain undiagnosed and untreated. Diabetes is a condition of full-blown blood glucose dysregulation in the body. Glucose, also referred to as "blood sugar" is the major hormone that supplies energy to all of the cells in the body. It helps to set the rate of metabolism, meaning the speed at which energy is burned by the body and afterward replenished for ongoing, everyday needs.

The process of glucose metabolism begins as foods containing this essential energy-producing hormone are consumed in the diet. One major organ that is especially dependent upon glucose to function properly is the brain but all other organs can also be affected by glucose imbalances (i.e. the kidneys, heart and liver), as can all other tissues in the body, including the nerves. When glucose reaches abnormally high levels, which is called "hyperglycemia", damage to these tissues and organs can begin to occur.

Common Diseases and Syndromes of Body Pain

This is also true of glucose levels that become abnormally low, which is called "hypoglycemia", meaning the body is being starved of this energy-regulating hormone. Both hyperglycemic and hypoglycemic episodes can occur with diabetes and if either is severe, they become a medical emergency and can also be life-threatening.

When the nerves are affected by glucose imbalances, a patient with diabetes or other conditions of blood glucose dysregulation may begin to experience one or more of the following symptoms that typically have a gradual onset.

- **Sensory Nerve Symptoms:**
- Tingling or burning sensations in the hands or feet
- Stabbing pains
- Numbness in toes, fingers or limbs
- A loss of sense in body positions, especially in the limbs
- **Motor Nerve Symptoms:**
- Weakness in the muscles
- Difficulty controlling muscle movements (ataxia)

- **Autonomic Nerve Symptoms:**
- Swelling in the extremities
- Difficulty sweating
- Blood pressure imbalances, especially upon first standing up
- Heart arrhythmias ...

Common Diseases and Syndromes of Body Pain

...
• Digestive problems
• Difficulty breathing (rare)

Hyperglycemia is the result of the body resisting the metabolizing effects of another important hormone produced by the pancreas called "insulin". This hormone is responsible for carrying glucose into the cells of the body and in regulating levels of it within body. One of the ways it does this is by clearing-out any excess amounts of glucose that enter the bloodstream via one's daily diet. When excessive amounts of fats are consumed (converted into glucose by the liver or into "glycogen" to be stored) and high levels of refined sugars are consumed (simple carbohydrates), the pancreas works excessively hard to clear these from the body. The liver aids in this process via a process called "gluconeogenesis".

A diet that is chronically abusive to this system or that in-essence overwhelms it, results in accumulation of fat and glucose in the body. Early stages of dysfunction in this process are referred to as "metabolic syndromes" or "pre-diabetic conditions". Obesity is a common indicator of developing metabolic problems, regardless of cause. In many cases, these can be reversed by improving one's diet and replacing simple carbohydrates with complex ones and by incorporating proper amounts of exercise into one's daily regimen.

Common Diseases and Syndromes of Body Pain

If hormone imbalances of other types are present (i.e. thyroid or sex hormone deficiencies), correcting these can be essential to correcting these problems with glucose dysregulation as well.

When full-blown diabetes occurs whether it is Type I (the genetic type with early onset usually during childhood) or Type II (later life onset, resulting from obesity, lack of exercise and improper diet), medical treatment becomes necessary in addition to lifestyle changes. Oral glucose regulating drugs may be prescribed or in more severe cases, a patient may require regular injections of insulin. Patients, who are successful in weight loss and in getting proper exercise, can actually diminish the need for treatments or possibly not require them at all at some point. It is however important that diabetic patients continue to monitor their glucose levels via a home blood test monitor and/or by regular checkups from their treating doctors.

The number of US citizens suffering from pre-diabetic conditions, is estimated by the American Diabetes Association to be approximately 57 million Americans. Medical research has strongly indicated that PN can develop with pre-diabetic conditions and so "prevention" via the previously described lifestyle changes/practices is vitally important.

Common Diseases and Syndromes of Body Pain

CHAPTER THREE

Other Systemic Diseases Associated with Development of PN

Diabetes, thyroid diseases and sex hormone imbalances have been mentioned in the previous two chapters but there are many other diseases that are of the inflammatory and/or autoimmune types that can also cause or contribute to the development of PN.

These include:

• Lupus
• Celiac Disease
• Rheumatoid Arthritis
• Sjogren's Syndrome
• Peripheral Artery Disease

Lupus: There are basically four types of lupus erythematosus (LE). The disease is also considered to be of the inflammatory and rheumatic type. Types of lupus erythematosus (LE) include "discoid" (round lesions and scarring affecting the skin), "neonatal" (present at birth), "drug-induced" (resulting from illegal drug-use or prescription ones) and "systemic" (multi-organ, tissues, blood vessels, nerves and cells).

15

Patients diagnosed with discoid LE, are at high risk for developing the systemic type. Many patients with LE go on to develop other autoimmune diseases as well, such as those affecting endocrine glands (i.e. thyroid, pancreas and adrenals) and rheumatoid arthritis.

Lupus Treatment: While there is no cure for LE, there are treatments designed to help relieve symptoms and to slow or halt the progression of the disease. Anti-inflammatory drugs may be recommended or prescribed depending on the strength needed. Some patients may only need over-the-counter drugs for inflammation and/or fever, such as aspirin or ibuprofen, while others may need those that are prescription-strength anti-inflammatory steroids (corticosteroids). Drugs that help to control immune system activity may also be prescribed as well as pain medications and hormone replacement therapies when needed.

Celiac Disease: An autoimmune condition of severe gluten intolerance that can cause digestive symptoms, malnutrition, anemia and damage to the digestive tract. Some medical sources are now of the opinion that "gluten sensitivity" can exist in patients, even when full-blown Celiac Disease is not present. For some people, especially those who are already suffering from other autoimmune diseases; their bodies begin to develop intolerances to things they eat that contain wheat, barley, rye and oats (gluten and related proteins).

Common Diseases and Syndromes of Body Pain

Their bodies began to recognize these foods as being harmful and their immune systems create antibodies to attack cells found in the lining of the small intestine that help break down gluten so that the body absorbs the nutrients from it. As a result, inflammation develops in the digestive tract and the person suffering the condition will begin to experience symptoms. The lack of nutrients being absorbed can result in damaged nerves over time if treatment is delayed.

Celiac Disease Treatment: The most important part of treatment for Celiac disease is to remove all products containing gluten from the diet. This would include the following gluten-containing food products: oats, wheat products, breads, cookies, cereals and beverages containing barely or malt. If inflammation in the small intestine is severe or not easily resolved by eliminating gluten from the diet, the treating doctor may prescribe a corticosteroid anti-inflammatory drug to reduce inflammation. Treatment will also include supplementing the patient with any nutrients or vitamins that have become low in their system due to past or ongoing mal-absorption of them. If damage to the small intestine occurs in a patient, medications to help with digestion and stomach upset may also be prescribed and rarely patients may need surgical removal of severely damaged areas of the small intestine.

Rheumatoid Arthritis: In the case of RA, the immune system recognizes components involving the areas of the body where bones attach to each other (joints) as threats in the body and sends out killer cells called "antibodies" to attack them. These natural tissues are mistakenly identified by the immune system as intruders or invaders that threaten bodily health. The joint-related tissues affected by RA include bones, cartilage, fibrous tissue, nerves and synovial fluid. This form of arthritis causes destruction of the joints over time and in some cases can also cause joints to become locked in place (fused) and immobile. It typically affects the small joints in the extremities (hands and feet) but can potentially affect any of the joints of the body. Over time RA can also cause inflammation in blood vessels (vasculitis).

Rheumatoid Arthritis Treatment: The goal for treating autoimmune arthritis is to control and alleviate symptoms being experienced and to slow the progression of the disease to prevent joint destruction, unnatural bone fusions and deformities. Patients with less severe inflammation may be prescribed milder types of anti-inflammatory drugs such as ibuprofen, indomethacin or naproxen. In more severe cases, prescription-strength anti-inflammatory medications may be required called "corticosteroids" which are steroids that mimic the inflammation moderating properties of the adrenal hormone "cortisol."

Common Diseases and Syndromes of Body Pain

Less common treatments used to treat more progressed cases of RA include the injection of "gold compounds" into the joints and imunno-suppressive drug therapies to slow-down over activity by the immune system. Additional drug therapies that may be used in some cases may include D-penicillamine, anti-malarial drugs, and sulfasalazine.

Sjogren's Syndrome (SS): An autoimmune, inflammatory disease that affects the fluid-producing and lubricating glands and tissues in the body. (SS) can co-exist with other types of autoimmune diseases and is especially common in people who suffer autoimmune thyroid diseases and rheumatoid arthritis. The severity of the disease varies among patients who have it and in some cases, it can become disabling. Sjogren's syndrome (pronounced "show-grins") affects the fluid producing ducts and glands of the body, as well as mucous membranes in the body. When a person has SS, the immune system has sent out killer cells, called antibodies, to attack these mechanisms of the body that produce lubricating fluids and membranes. This, results in these fluids and membranes becoming dry, so that the parts of the body that contain them may also become inflamed and/or damaged, including the nerves.

Sjogren's Syndrome Treatment: There is no specific treatment for this autoimmune disease and so the treatment is to reduce the effects of the bodily symptoms it causes. For patients who experience dry eyes, doctors may prescribe synthetic tear solutions or pharmaceutical grade eye drops to help keep the eyes lubricated. The same is true of patients with dry sinuses; nose drops may be prescribed to help moisturize the dry tissues in the nose and sinus passages. Patients with joint pain may be prescribed medications to treat arthritic and rheumatic symptoms. For those patients with chronic and severe inflammation, a corticosteroid may be prescribed to reduce the inflammation, such as the commonly prescribed anti-inflammatory called "Prednisone."

Peripheral Artery Disease (PAD): Is a condition in which the arteries that distribute blood-flow to different parts of the body become hardened, narrowed or blocked. As tissues and nerves are starved of proper blood flow, symptoms of pain and muscle weakness begin to develop. PAD commonly develops in the arteries that supply blood to the pelvis and the legs and may be restricted to the limbs or may affect many areas of the body simultaneously, including the heart. The condition is more common in people who have diabetes, who smoke or who have reached their elder years of age. In severe cases, body tissues experience permanent death and must be amputated from the body.

Common Diseases and Syndromes of Body Pain

Some patients with the disease lose their ability to walk and may be at increased risk for heart attack or stroke.

Peripheral Artery Disease Treatment: Treatments for PAD are directed at relieving symptoms of pain in the legs via over-the-counter or prescription-strength pain medications. If arteries have become narrowed, drugs are available that can help to open the arteries and to increase blood-flow through them. Blood-thinning medications may also be prescribed to help accomplish this.

If high cholesterol is the cause of obstructed arteries, medications that help lower the cholesterol may be prescribed, as well as those that can treat any hypertension that might also be present in a patient, which can contribute to damaged arteries. Patients who smoke may be referred to programs that help them quit or to medications to curb their addiction, while weaning off of tobacco-smoking (a strong contributor to symptoms of PAD).

PN that results from the health disorders described above or from other underlying chronic diseases, such as AIDS and types of lymphoma cancers, can be significantly improved by treating them as optimally as possible.

Some patients do however; require treatment specifically for their PN symptoms, as they await improvement or recovery from their disease or for permanent nerve damage that has occurred. Treatments that are specifically directed at PN symptoms will be further discussed in chapters that follow.

CHAPTER FOUR

Viruses that Cause or Contribute to PN

A number of viruses have been found to be triggers for symptoms of PN. Some of these cause gradual, progressive symptoms of nerve damage and dysfunction (chronic), while others or even the same viruses can cause a sudden and severe onset of them (acute). In some cases the severity of the PN following a viral infection is dependent upon how severe an infection is or in how well the infected person's immune system is functioning during and following a contracted viral infection.

These PN causing viruses can include those following, as listed below.

- * Cytomegalovirus
- * Epstein-Barr
- * Varicella Zoster
- Hepatitis Viruses A, B, C, D, and E
- Campylobacter Jejuni (actually in the "bacteria" family and rare)

The viruses listed on the previous page, including *hepatitis* which encompasses several sub-types, can be triggers for a neurological condition called Guillain-Barre syndrome (GBS). The three viruses included in the list with asterisks beside them (*) are from the "herpes" family and a majority of the general population will carry them in their bodies, once contracting them, life-long but most do not suffer ongoing symptoms after initial infections by them during childhood. The viruses will usually remain dormant and benign but can reactivate in imunno-compromised individuals (in those with deficient immune function).

Another term for GBS and the peripheral nerve symptoms and/or damage, resulting from autoimmune reactions, following viral infections or due to other causes that activate auto-antibodies to attack nerves is "Chronic Inflammatory Demyelinating Polyneuropathy" (CIDP). The "polyneuropathy" aspect of the term, refers to the fact that multiple nerves are being affected simultaneously. When only one nerve is affected by a disease or damage that occurs to it, the term "mononeuropathy" is used.

The onset of CIDP can manifest with something as simple as a hand or foot that drops due to a lack of motor-nerve impulses carried to the muscles of them.

Other patients may experience the onset of severe pain in their feet and legs or in other parts of their body, due to sensory nerve involvement and this may be accompanied by an overall body-weakness and fatigue.

The **Cytomegalovirus**, also referred-to as "Human Herpesvirus 5" (HCMV), may initially affect the salivary glands in the body but often goes on the cause a systemic infection (body-wide) in susceptible individuals. People at risk for serious or even life-threatening responses to an HCMV infection, are typically those who have co-existing diseases affecting the immune system, those who have undergone organ transplants and newborn infants.

Campylobacter Jejuni, is a bacterium that can be contracted through drinking water or food that is not properly purified or handled under clean conditions (food borne infection), leading to gastrointestinal infections in humans. It is becoming highly recognized as a major cause of Guillain-Barre syndrome, worldwide.

Varicella Zoster, is a virus that initially causes two medical conditions called "shingles" (more common in adults) and "chicken pox" (more common in children), while the **Epstein-Barr virus** can first manifest as a condition called "mononucleosis" (the kissing disease).

Common Diseases and Syndromes of Body Pain

These viruses have also been associated with causing GBS/CIDP in susceptible individuals and in some cases may be due to their immune systems having become weakened or compromised due to other chronic or autoimmune diseases.

For reasons yet fully understood by medical research science, these viruses can lead to an immune system reaction, in which the "myelin", a material that covers the outside of the nerves, acting as a protective sheath for them, comes under attack by auto-antibodies, that mistakenly recognize them as intruders and enemies to the body.

These killer immune cells begin to attack this essential part of the peripheral nervous system as an enemy in the body and may do-so, even after a particular viral infection has diminished or is no longer active.

It is possible that this misguided immune activity is an over-reactive response by the immune system, to fully eradicate these viruses from the body and in the process of doing so, results in damage to nerves that become exposed and unprotected over time.

Treating GBS/CIDP

Conditions of PN caused by the autoimmune and inflammatory components that have been described may include the administration of a prescribed steroid anti-inflammatory drug (corticosteroid), by a qualified physician. In some cases this type medication, commonly prescribed via the brand-name "Prednisone", will alleviate and reverse GBS/CIDP, without the need for further treatments. This may depend on how advanced the condition has become.

For those patients with severe symptoms needing more advanced treatments, a treating doctor may refer them for a therapy called "Intravenous immunoglobulin" (IVIG). This treatment consists of administering this plasma protein, intravenously at regular intervals of every few weeks, until the patient's own immune system becomes better-charged with healthy antibodies that help them to recover from their disease.

IVIG has also been suggested by some medical experts, to be beneficial in helping to reduce inflammation levels as well. In some cases however, both IVIG and corticosteroid therapies may be administered.

The symptoms of GBS/CIDP can be treated successfully and in many cases completely reversed. Treatments for peripheral nerve disease symptoms will be further addressed in chapters FIVE and SIX that immediately follow.

CHAPTER FIVE

Nutritional Deficiencies that Lead to PN

The nutritional deficiencies that are listed below, each have the potential to negatively affect the peripheral nervous system. The treatments for these is simply to replace the missing nutrient via prescribed oral or intravenous therapies that bring the deficient levels back up to proper normal values. Symptoms in addition to potential neurological ones are also listed beside each nutrient shown below.

Vitamin A Deficiency – neurological symptoms, tiredness, stunted growth, insomnia, thick oily skin, immune dysfunction, night vision impairment, weight loss, dry hair

Vitamin B12 Deficiency – anemia, numbness, burning and tingling in the legs, arms, feet and hands, loss of muscle coordination and muscle weakness, ringing in the ears, dizziness and loss of balance, slowed or erratic reflexes, irritability and confusion, anxiety and depression (neuro-psychiatric)

Common Diseases and Syndromes of Body Pain

Vitamin C Deficiency - irritability, joint pain, tooth loss, fatigue, gum disease, depression, easy bruising, slowed wound healing, peripheral nerve symptoms

Vitamin D Deficiency - anxiety, osteomalacia (soft bones), bone loss, rickets (bone deformity in children), excessive sweating, burning or tingling sensations in mouth, diarrhea, inability to sleep, nearsightedness

Vitamin E Deficiency - slowed reflexes, lost sense of position, lost sense of vibration, loss of red blood cells, unsteady gait, ataxia, peripheral nerve pain, loss of muscle strength

Vitamin K Deficiency – inability for blood to clot, excessive bleeding, lack of proper blood supply to nerves

Biotin (B7) Deficiency – clumsiness in muscles, insomnia, myopathy, skin rash and dryness, opthalmopathy, hair that falls out, neurological deficits

Calcium Deficiency - depression, inability to sleep, irritability, bone loss, heart arrhythmias, periodontal disease, rickets, tooth loss, dry nails, stomach cramps, hysteria and hallucinations, peripheral neuropathy

Common Diseases and Syndromes of Body Pain

Chromium Deficiency - glucose dysregulation, type II diabetes, anxiety, fatigue, nerve damage from chronic glucose imbalance

Copper Deficiency - depression, diarrhea, tiredness, brittle bones, hair that falls out, hyperthyroidism, weak muscles, anemia, arterial artery damage, lack of nourishment to nerves

Deficiencies of Essential Fatty Acids - immune dysfunction, inability to conceive, low sperm count, slowed wound healing, heavy menstrual cycles and PMS, acne, rash and dry skin, gall bladder stones, liver damage, diarrhea, brittle hair and hair loss, neurological disease

Folic acid (B9) Deficiency - headaches, inability to sleep, low appetite and weight loss, fetal deformity, psychosis, breathing difficulties, muscle weakness, anemia, low mood and apathy, diarrhea, tiredness, peripheral nerve dysfunction

Iron Deficiency - depression, vertigo, tiredness, headaches, sore tongue, mouth sores, anemia, brittle nails, dementia, constipation, lack of blood supply to nerves

Common Diseases and Syndromes of Body Pain

Magnesium Deficiency - hyperactivity, inability to sleep, nervousness, muscular dysfunction and myopathy, restlessness, weakness, anxiety, dementia, heart disease, nerve dysfunction

Manganese Deficiency - hypercholesterolemia, glucose intolerance, hearing problems, clumsy muscles, tinnitus, atherosclerosis, dizziness and vertigo, nerve damage due to lack of blood supply and glucose to nerves

Niacin (B3) Deficiency - diarrhea, mood disorder, tiredness, irritability, weight loss and loss of appetite, short-term memory loss, myopathy, nausea, skin lesions and dermopathy, bad breath, canker sores, confusion, depression, dermatitis, neurological disease

Pantothenic acid (B5) Deficiency - hair loss, immune impairment, insomnia, irritability, hypotension, muscle cramps, nausea, lack of coordination, abdominal cramps, peripheral neuropathy in feet, depression, eczema, tiredness

Potassium Deficiency - tiredness, hyperglycemia, elevated cholesterol, insomnia, dementia, myopathy, anxiety, hyporeflexia, oily skin, constipation, depression, edema, excessive thirst, nerve dysfunction

Common Diseases and Syndromes of Body Pain

Pyridoxine (B6) Deficiency - tiredness, slowed wound healing, irritability, low appetite, hair loss, mouth sores, nausea, acne, anemia, joint pain, opthalmopathy, depression, dizziness, oily face, peripheral neuropathy (Deficiency in this vitamin is fairly rare but can occur in cases of chronic alcoholism.)

Riboflavin (B2) Deficiency – peripheral neuropathies (numb hands or feet, loss of sensation, shock or vibration sensations), seizure, eye-sensitivity to light, insomnia and tiredness, weakness, blurry vision, cataracts, low mood, dry-inflamed skin, dizziness and vertigo, hair falling out, eye inflammation, mouth sores, nervousness and irritability

Selenium Deficiency - pancreatitis, indigestion, immune dysfunction, liver dysfunction, low sperm count, stunted growth, elevated cholesterol, increased risk of cancer, lack of nerve function

Thiamin (B1) Deficiency - low appetite and weight loss, loss of short-term memory, anxiety, peripheral neuropathy, increased pain sensitivity, lack of coordination, weak muscles, dementia, constipation, indigestion, irritability (Deficiency of this vitamin is also called "beriberi disease" but is rare with exception to countries that eat polished rice almost exclusively.)

Common Diseases and Syndromes of Body Pain

Zinc Deficiency - elevated cholesterol, immune dysfunction, erectile dysfunction, irritability, malaise, low appetite, lack of ability to taste, low stomach acid (hypochlorhydria), low sperm count, short-term memory loss, partial loss of nighttime vision, psychosis, white areas in the middle of fingernails, slowed wound healing, acne, amnesia, malaise, dry hair and nails, delayed puberty, depressed mood, diarrhea, dry skin rashes, tiredness, stunted growth, loss of hair, neurological deficits

Iodine Deficiency – under-active thyroid gland, weight gain, cretinism (neonatal and congenital hypothyroidism), tiredness, joint and muscle aches, peripheral nerve entrapment from myxedema (tissue swelling)

Common Diseases and Syndromes of Body Pain

CHAPTER SIX

Directly Addressing Pain Symptoms of PN

As has been discussed in the previous chapters, a major aspect of treatment for peripheral neuropathies of any type is to address any potential underlying causes of them, whether these are endocrine gland imbalances, nutritional deficiencies or chronic inflammatory and autoimmune diseases. Correction of these medical problems, can greatly contribute to improvement of PN symptoms. Since most of these have been covered previously, this chapter will be mainly dedicated to treatments that are designed at specifically relieving and possibly alleviating PN pain symptoms, in addition to treatments directed at underlying causes.

Drugs that Treat Nerve Pain

There are many types of pain relief medications, including both the prescribed types and those that can be purchased over-the-counter. There are however three classes of drugs that are specifically directed at relieving nerve pain, which include the following types and brands.

• **Over-The-Counter Drugs:**
• Acetaminophen
• Aspirin ...

Common Diseases and Syndromes of Body Pain

...

- ibuprofen
- Naproxen

- **Antidepressants:**

- Tricyclic Antidepressants (TCA's) – (i.e. Types: Amitriptyline and Nortriptiline)
- Selective Serotonin Reuptake Inhibitors (SSRI) – (i.e. Brands: Paxil, Prozac, Zoloft)

- **Anticonvulsants:**

- Gabapentin
- Carbamazepine
- Felbamate
- Valproic Acid
- Clonazepam
- Phenytoin

In severe cases of nerve pain, that fails to improve with pain medications, patients may be referred for "nerve block treatments", which consist of a series of injections into the areas of pain, using a substance such as alcohol or phenol (carbolic acid) to interrupt pain signals from damaged nerves. The injections are given at regular intervals, to help with ongoing pain.

Common Diseases and Syndromes of Body Pain

Nerve Entrapment Therapies

When pain is referred from a nerve that is being pinched (nerve entrapment), treatments will be directed at relieving the pressure on the affected nerves. Some nerve entrapments cause significant pain, such as those affecting the "sciatic nerve" (a large nerve that runs from the back, into the legs and feet), the "median nerve" (affecting the wrists and hands) and the posterior tibial nerve (affecting the feet and toes). Treatments may include surgical procedures, massage and chiropractic therapies, temperature applications (ice packs or heating pads) and isolation, meaning a period of restricted or non-movement of limbs or other body-parts that contain the entrapped nerves. In some cases, nerve-stimulation devices are used in attempt to stimulate proper impulses from nerves that have been affected by long-term entrapment.

Conclusion:

Peripheral Neuropathies are common conditions that can cause significant pain, muscle weakness and disability to its sufferers but treatments are available. Certainly a healthy lifestyle is also instrumental to improving the symptoms of PN.

This would nclude a healthy diet, carefully undertaken and regulated exercise and methods of stress-reduction. It is my hope that the preceding chapters of this book have provided a general educational resource for those seeking information on treating this illness, which can help to gain its sufferers, an improved quality of life and an increased sense of well-being.

(END - SECTION ONE)

SECTION TWO:

A Complete Look at CFS and Fibromyalgia

The Syndromes of Fatigue and Body Pain

TABLE OF CONTENTS

Common Diseases and Syndromes of Body Pain

INTRODUCTION

Chronic Fatigue Syndrome and Fibromyalgia affect millions of Americans and many millions more worldwide. The Debilitating fatigue and joint/muscle pain these syndromes cause can seriously reduce the quality-of-life for those who experience them. Aspects of these illnesses can include the following.

• Viral, fungal and bacterial components

• hormonal and nutritional deficiencies

• adrenal fatigue (low cortisol and/or DHEA levels)

Chronic Fatigue Syndrome and Fibromyalgia are real illnesses recognized by the U.S. National Institutes of Health and other World Health Organizations. While they are separately recognized illnesses, they have 75% crossover similarities. It is my hope that this book will provide an informative general educational resource for readers wishing to learn more about these very real, life-changing illnesses.

Common Diseases and Syndromes of Body Pain

CHAPTER ONE

The Symptoms of Chronic Fatigue Syndrome and Fibromyalgia

Since many symptoms of CFS and Fibromyalgia are in-common with both syndromes, the symptom list that follows will be an equal possibility for being experienced with both syndromes. With the two major characteristic symptoms that distinguish between the two syndromes being "fatigue" (CFS) and "body pain" (Fibromyalgia). Both can be present in each illness but if one or the other is prominent, this helps to distinguish between them.

• Fatigue (ongoing and following exertion)

• Joint/muscle aches & tender points (with the absence of redness or swelling of joints)

• Neurological symptoms (i.e. headaches, tremors, dizziness and sensory changes)

• Emotional symptoms (i.e. anxiety and/or depression)

• Cognitive problems (i.e. difficulty concentrating and short-term memory loss)

The following two stories are fictitious examples, written by me – the author, to serve as examples of how one might discover that they are suffering from CFS and/or Fibromyalgia.

Common Diseases and Syndromes of Body Pain

Fictitious Scenario for Fibromyalgia:

Jane Doe says:
"When I was in my mid thirties, I started having some joint pain that started in my knees and I thought it was from doing too much gardening on my hands and knees. I didn't think much about it until I noticed more muscle stiffness and aches as months and years went by. One morning I woke up and I felt this stiffness throughout my body and began to wonder if I might have some kind of arthritis affecting me. I started taking pain relief - over the counter medicines which helped some but the muscle pain continued to worsen overall and after a while I was taking the highest dose of brand name pain medicines you could buy off the shelf. I knew then it was time to see a doctor and ask about tests for arthritis.

The doctor I ended up with told me my problem was just from aging and going through the menopause age but I knew it was far more serious and I asked him if tests for arthritis might be a good idea. He told me that without any joint swelling or redness around my joints, these type tests were of no purpose. I went home that day greatly disappointed because my hope was in being prescribed something to help with the pain that had spread all over by body. I was watching a television documentary about a man who went through almost exactly what I was going through and it got my attention when they diagnosed him with fibromyalgia.

Common Diseases and Syndromes of Body Pain

I made a new appointment with a different doctor whose specialty was diabetes but who was known for being more thorough with patients. He listened to my story and started a physical exam of me and he started to press his finger in different areas of my muscles and this caused remarkable pain on some of these spots. He didn't even have to ask me when I had pain because I would jump and wince when some of these spots were pressed against. He had an expression of recognition on his face at that point and when I questioned him he said that it was almost certain I had fibromyalgia because I had at least 11 tender spots around different joints in my body.

I was relieved in one sense and scared in another. He had me get blood tests for arthritis and autoimmune problems and these were negative I had a mild elevation in inflammation shown on the test results and a mildly high creatinine kinase blood level which indicated mild muscle damage with a small degree of inflammation. He told me that many fibromyalgia patients have no positive lab findings but that my physical exam and medical history was certain for my having it. My doctor is treating me with analgesic drugs for pain and inflammation and he has me on a low dose of anti-seizure medication which also helps with pain. I may also have an antidepressant added to my treatment if these other drugs are not completely successful in relieving the pain. At this point I'm just hoping for the best with the treatment I'm already on."

Common Diseases and Syndromes of Body Pain

Fictitious Scenario for Chronic Fatigue Syndrome:

John Doe says:
"As a college student in the 1990s, I woke up one morning and literally, that day found I was totally exhausted and drained of energy. This continued for months, in fact after six months the fatigue was still not letting up. I just barely functioned enough to complete my required studies and tests. I felt so drained after cramming for tests or taking them that it took me two days to rest up from them. I went to the campus clinic and was told I had depression but I knew better. My mom set an appointment for me with her doctor and he performed tests on me for 3 months and I mean for everything under the sun that might be wrong with me. The test findings that stuck out were my virus counts which were through the roof. I had an Epstein-Barr virus number in the 100s and an HV6 virus count also in the 100s. The doctor said this showed that my immune system was not functioning normally and he started me on immune boosting drugs and vitamins. I improved about 40% after a little over four months and have since improved about 60% and hoping for more improvement. Chronic Fatigue Syndrome is real and let no one tell you otherwise. My doctor told me that some people heal from it while others only recover partially and have symptoms for many years. He assured me that younger people who get CFS recover better and more completely than do middle age people and older."

Common Diseases and Syndromes of Body Pain

CHAPTER TWO

Conditions That Cause Mild Adrenal Insufficiency

Adrenal insufficiency is a condition in which the adrenal glands do not produce enough hormones to aid in regulating the body's metabolism, stress coping, controlling inflammation and sexual functioning. The main adrenal hormone that becomes low with this condition is "cortisol," and when low levels are detected in a person, it is sometimes referred to as "hypocortisolemia". Full blown adrenal insufficiency is referred to as "Addison's Disease." There are, however, milder forms of adrenal dysfunction as listed below.

Post Traumatic Stress Disorder. This condition, abbreviated PTSD, is a traumatic stress-caused condition that is also considered to be an anxiety disorder. People experience the onset of this disorder as a result of severe traumatizing experiences, such as car accidents, acts of violence that are perpetrated upon them, the sudden loss of a loved one or having been in active combat during wartime. The severe shock caused to the body from such incidents can cause the glands regulating adrenal hormone output to become "blunted", meaning they begin to function at a sub-normal level.

While their adrenal hormones may remain within normal limits, they will be at lowest normal (borderline low), which causes them to have an inability to cope with stressors.

Research studies on PTSD that are published by reputable medical groups (including the U.S. National Institutes of Health) state that low cortisol levels found in patients with this disorder contributes to their symptoms of anxiety, insomnia and flashbacks, meaning they may mentally relive their traumatic experiences repeatedly. In controlled test studies, using cortisol supplementation to treat PTSD patients, results showed that symptoms were reduced significantly by carefully monitored physiological dosing to increase their level of the low stress hormone.

Chronic Fatigue Syndrome (CFS). This condition has also been found to cause a low level of the stress hormone cortisol evidenced by analyzing the blood and urine cortisol levels in people who experience the illness. Research studies on CFS have repeatedly confirmed this fact and have also found that patients report that they were experiencing chronic or sudden severe stress just before the onset of the illness. This would mean that CFS is very possibly also a stress-related condition that causes the adrenal hormone regulating glands in the body to become blunted.

Common Diseases and Syndromes of Body Pain

The U.S. National Institutes of Health released a report in October of 1996, in which they found through a controlled study, that cortisol supplementation/replacement in patients with CFS had a benefit but was found to be short-lived. Afterward, some patients began experiencing a more severe form of adrenal suppression, meaning it caused a worsening of their adrenal insufficiency after a few weeks on the cortisol replacement drug.

Fibromyalga Syndrome (FMS). Being very similar to CFS, Fibromyalgia also has chronic fatigue as a major symptom. The aspect that sets this illness apart from CFS is the widespread body pain that is not found to be as prominent in CFS patients. Despite this fact, researchers studying both illnesses have found them to have 75% crossover similarities. This includes the fact that FMS patients often report chronic stress as being a factor in their development of the illness.

A number of research studies have also found cortisol levels to be low in FMS patients and controlled trials of cortisol supplementation have been conducted to determine if there would be a benefit for these patients. The findings were similar to those found when supplementing CFS patients with cortisol hormone replacement.

While some patients improved, the long-term risks for using the drug (i.e. adrenal suppression) did not merit establishing it as a medically recognized treatment for FMS.

Adrenal Fatigue. This sub-clinical form of adrenal insufficiency is still not recognized widely by the medical community, although certain types of doctors recognize the disorder, including MDs who practice holistic treatments, Naturopaths and Osteopathic Physicians.

With this condition which is also referred to as "low adrenal reserves" and "adrenal exhaustion", many of the symptoms found in CFS and FMS are not present, including joint and muscle pain and other inflammatory problems in the body.

Adrenal Fatigue is strictly a condition causing mild to moderate fatigue and reduced stress tolerance. Some medical sources are stating that adrenal fatigue that is prolonged and not treated, through proper rest, improved diet, adrenal boosting natural supplements and reducing contributing stressors, may result in the condition becoming a precursor (a pre-condition) to CFS and FMS.

While the conditions listed above are commonly found to cause mild adrenal insufficiency, other conditions can also be a cause or contributing factor, including other chronic and inflammatory diseases that contribute to increased stress levels in the body.

CHAPTER THREE

The Role of Adrenal Fatigue in Illnesses

Many Doctors only recognize the most severe form of adrenal hypo-function called Addison's' Disease or full blown adrenal insufficiency and they base whether or not a patient has this potentially life-threatening form, via the "ACTH Stimulation Test".

The problem is that many people have a less severe form called adrenal fatigue or adrenal exhaustion and though these patients nearly always pass the ACTH Stimulation Test, they still have inadequate adrenal hormone levels that show up clearly on lab tests and though it is not life-threatening, it still causes concerning symptoms that can seriously affect quality of life.

The National Institutes of Health, while studying Chronic Fatigue Syndrome, found "low cortisol" to be a factor in it as well and in one of these studies, they made this statement; "Doctors have long known that even subtle deficiencies in cortisol can be associated with lethargy and fatigue."

The "NIAMS" (arthritis etc...) Department of the National Institutes of Health also recognizes low cortisol in Fibromyalgia.

Common Diseases and Syndromes of Body Pain

Other studies they've published on the PubMed/National Libraries of Medicine website, also recognize low cortisol in PTSD (Post Traumatic Stress Disorders). The fact is that adrenal fatigue can be a factor in these and other chronic diseases/syndromes but other times is stress-related or not related to anything specific.

The most important thing, if you feel you may have adrenal fatigue, is to be tested for it because other hormone imbalances and illnesses cause similar symptoms. Some pharmacies are now carrying saliva hormone testing kits, including ones that test adrenal hormones (cortisol), so you may want to check for the availability of these in your area. If they are not available locally, one can order them online using the search term "adrenal hormone saliva test kits".

The passion I have in the area of adrenal fatigue, besides experiencing it myself, as part of CFS and thyroid disease is the fact that far too many studies and reputable organizations recognize it. This includes the "Fibro & Fatigue Centers", located in 15 states that are staffed by Board Certified MDs from just about every field of medicine. This plus the fact that there are U.S. Government health studies that have also concluded that there are low-cortisol syndromes or well established sub-clinical forms of adrenal hypo-function, that could all be referred to under the term; "adrenal fatigue".

CHAPTER FOUR

Cortisol & DHEA Supplements for Adrenal Fatigue

Over the past four years, I have written a lot on the subject of mild hypo-cortisolism that is found in different conditions, that for lack of another well-established term, we call "adrenal fatigue" but it is often during the research I'm doing at any given time for articles etc..., that I find often, that many in the medical community, still do not recognize mild forms of adrenal insufficiency and they do not believe that adrenal fatigue syndromes exist.

I actually hope Doctors or knowledgeable people of any type will make a suggestion for a name that doesn't come across as bogus and at the same time, if they don't believe sub-clinical forms of adrenal hypo-cortisolism exist, to also explain why all of the research articles that describe it, are somehow all collectively wrong on the subject.

The majority of adrenal fatigue patients will at times have snap-shot readings that are normal, when blood tested for cortisol levels and they will also pass the ACTH Stimulation Test (confirms or rules out full blown adrenal insufficiency) and is why it is recommended to get multiple readings throughout the day, via saliva cortisol testing for milder forms of adrenal hypo-cortisolism.

Common Diseases and Syndromes of Body Pain

When I had the ACTH Stimulation Test performed on me, my cortisol reading was about mid-range on the baseline reading however, I was anxious before and during the test and it's better to get cortisol rhythm of multi-readings during a normal activity day. Even though I had a normal baseline on that ACTH Stimulation Test, I also had a 24 hour urinary test through an Endocrinologist's Office and my cortisol averaged "10.7", with normal range at the lab being <119 for males ages 18 and above. To be in the middle of that one (mid-range), I would have had to have a result of about a 50 or 60 and my Dr. admitted it was a very low reading for a 24 hour urine cortisol test. This confirmed I didn't have true, full-blown adrenal insufficiency but that I did have a serious case of adrenal fatigue.

In research articles, where patients with different diseases, are found to have low cortisol levels, the medical investigators are usually referring to "low cortisol" as being in the low-normal range, so is low compared to "controls" and low compared to normal subjects. They even give the number differences, calling them "significant" even when the difference is only 2 or 3 points lower than normal subjects have. One statement the NIH makes in their Centers For Disease Control study of CFS, that has always stuck with me is this one; "Doctors have long known that even subtle deficiencies in cortisol is associated with lethargy and fatigue" (Oct, 1996).

Common Diseases and Syndromes of Body Pain

I've lately come more to the conclusion that I've suspected from the beginning of researching on adrenal fatigue, that supplementing with DHEA, will help low DHEA levels but usually doesn't help with low cortisol. Maybe in some patients it does help to raise cortisol, once the circle of conversion goes completely around but there's conflicting info about DHEA out there. What will help the adrenals to produce more cortisol, are vitamins that support adrenal function, rest and adequate sleep and if needed, the safe and cautious use of licorice extract and adrenal glandular extracts.

Some Doctors also sometimes prescribe; pregnenolone to adrenal fatigue patients or other combinations of hormones. A lot of medical resources say that the majority of women can safely take 25mg or less of DHEA and there is very low risk of it causing their androgen levels (male hormones) to go too high and men are supposed to be able to take up to 50mg safely.

I don't feel DHEA would suppress cortisol to a significant degree at these doses but the point is that they also might not help raise cortisol, so that taking it alone, could cause more of a DHEA to cortisol ratio imbalance. This isn't true of people who have low DHEA but normal cortisol levels because DHEA is all they need in these cases.

The Journal of Pharmacology has a research article that states that patients with Crohn's Disease and Lupus, are one example of low DHEA, that when supplemented, improves symptoms of these diseases but DHEA can become low for other reasons as well.

The "American Psychiatric Association", made a statement in the "American Journal of Psychiatry", in a research test that was conducted by 3 psychiatrists and 6 MDs. They stated that supplementing Post Traumatic Stress Disorder patients (PTSD) with low-dose cortical can help them because they found that the low cortisol found in this condition, is a major factor in symptoms. This study, which didn't go overboard with the dosing of cortisol, like others have, such as those experimenting with cortisol supplementing in CFS patients, had more favorable results that are promising for future studies.

There are now studies reported by the major medical research publishing groups that show that CFS patients did improve with lower-dose cortisol treatment. These studies are newer than the ones where they reported "adrenal suppression" and other adverse effects at higher dose treatment. Cortisol replacement therapy is only available by prescription, by a licensed medical professional but hopefully as more research is done, they will find a safe dose that will help treat adrenal fatigue type syndromes.

CHAPTER FIVE

Epstein-Barr Virus and Chronic Fatigue Syndrome

One major virus that other NIH studies have concluded as being highly associated with CFS, which also has low cortisol as a feature, is the Epstein-Barr Virus which causes mononucleosis. I had a severe case of mononucleosis as a kid, at about age-10 and have always believed there is a connection of it, to both my thyroid disease and CFS.

When I was optimized on HRT but continued to have symptoms, some that were not typical of thyroid, including;

• severe post exertion malaise

• swollen neck lymph nodes

• orthostatic hypotension (dizzy when first standing)

• chemical sensitivities

I decided to get tested for EBV. I had read so much about research that suggests the possibility that EBV like others in the herpes virus family, can flare-up in persons with a compromised or deficient immune system (immune dysfunction). My EBV/IGG result was "218" with the normal range being <20 (less than twenty).

Common Diseases and Syndromes of Body Pain

This means my EBV count was more than 10 times the normal cut-off range.

While a large percent of the population tests positive for EBV (statistics estimate 80%), titers as high as mine are not common, unless a person is actually experiencing active mononucleosis. In my case, I feel the EBV has a connection to both my Hashimoto's Thyroiditis and CFS. The NIH also has research published on the PubMed website that associates EBV with autoimmune thyroiditis.

The Epstein-Barr Virus (EBV) subject is one of real interest to me, especially since searching and researching on the subject. I found lots of medical studies that associate EBV with lots of conditions and diseases not the least of which is Chronic Fatigue Syndrome/CFS. A few of these studies state that in people with deficiencies in their immune systems, the virus can "reactivate" (re-surge in phases) and also "replicate" (increase in phases). Not many doctors recognize these facts but they are true non-the-less and EBV has been linked to causing autoimmune diseases as well, such as autoimmune thyroid diseases.

In my opinion, EBV has been active in my system since having my having mononucleosis as a child. I also believe it is responsible for my autoimmune thyroid disease (Hashimoto's thyroiditis). Another interesting fact is sub-clinical to moderate thyroid hormone deficiency being found commonly in people with CFS.

Common Diseases and Syndromes of Body Pain

My lymph glands in my neck swell as well and feel mildly sore, in phases and have at least a mild swelling in them all of the time. My CFS symptoms also flare in phases and these can be more severe when I work extra hard or experience increased stress.

Here are quotes/links I find interesting on this subject:

Research quote – Oxford Journals:

"Reactivation of EBV infection is a common finding in immunocompromised individuals."
Research link>
http://ndt.oxfordjournals.org/cgi/content/abstract/12/10/2099

Research Quote – U.S. NIH:

"Although the symptoms of infectious mononucleosis usually resolve in 1 or 2 months, EBV remains dormant or latent in a few cells in the throat and blood for the rest of the person's life. Periodically, the virus can reactivate and is commonly found in the saliva of infected persons. This reactivation usually occurs without symptoms of illness....It is important to note that symptoms related to infectious mononucleosis caused by EBV infection seldom last for more than 4 months. When such an illness lasts more than 6 months, it is frequently called chronic EBV infection.

Common Diseases and Syndromes of Body Pain

However, valid laboratory evidence for continued active EBV infection is seldom found in these patients. The illness should be investigated further to determine if it meets the criteria for chronic fatigue syndrome, or CFS. This process includes ruling out other causes of chronic illness or fatigue."

Research link>>
http://www.cdc.gov/ncidod/diseases/ebv.htm (U.S. National Institutes of Health - Centers for Disease Control – reprints allowed for public education purposes.)

More in regard to the connection of EBV to both CFS and Fibromyalgia will be included in Chapter Seven.

CHAPTER SIX

My Own Diagnosis of Thyroid Disease, CFS and Adrenal Fatigue

One of the reasons I wish to include a chapter on my personal story is because of my thyroid disease aspect. Medical sources, including the National Institutes of Health (U.S.) have published medical research that strongly associates thyroid diseases, especially the autoimmune types, to Fibromyalgia.

There are also many thyroid patients who experience co-morbid CFS or a mix of both CFS and Fibromyalgia. One such person is well known Thyroid Patient Advocate Mary Shomon, who has written a book, as a result of experiencing these syndromes co-morbid to her thyroid disease, entitled "Living Well with Chronic Fatigue Syndrome and Fibromyalgia".

My ongoing battle with adrenal fatigue began to manifest even before I experienced the obvious onset of Hashimoto's/Hypothyroidism in early 2003. I began to notice months previous to diagnosis that my tolerance for stress and my recuperative abilities, to spring back from hard physical activity, illnesses, excessive stressors etc.., was slowly diminishing. When my hypothyroid disease kicked in, the adrenal fatigue hit a peak of severity and the combination of the two really threw me for a loop.

Common Diseases and Syndromes of Body Pain

When Chronic Disease is Left Untreated

The first Doctors I went to didn't investigate to find the thyroid disease and I was not being treated for it, so in the mean time I had to push myself incredibly hard just to keep going. I also had an extremely stressful job in property management at that time.

Finally at one point, the adrenal fatigue turned into severe "adrenal exhaustion" and I experienced a strange viral type illness that left me with severe hives (these resolved) and swollen neck lymph-nodes that are swollen to this day! This is also when my chemical sensitivities became much worse to caffeine chocolate, alcohol and stimulants of any kind. In other words I had developed increased Multiple Chemical Sensitivities (MCS).

I finally demanded blood tests and as a result, was treated for diagnosed-hypothyroidism but the adrenal fatigue remained, re-occurring in flares of symptoms. Over time, I learned the difference between the symptoms of adrenal fatigue/exhaustion and thyroid symptoms.

With adrenal exhaustion, I experience severe post-exertion malaise and it can take a couple of days sometimes to recuperate from hard physical activity.

My CFS and Abnormal TSH Level

In the year 2006, my blood lab results, to monitor my thyroid hormone therapy, including TSH, T-4 and Free T-3 (thyroid function tests), were not jiving or correlating with each other. My TSH, at just below 0.2 (normal range 0.3 to 5.0), did not match up with the thyroid hormone levels which were also low. Usually a low TSH will mean high readings of the thyroid hormones or "hyperthyroidism". Patients taking Armour Thyroid (brand of T-4/T-3 thyroid med I take) do commonly have a somewhat low T-4 level but usually not flagged below normal and a below normal TSH usually means over-treatment with thyroid medication but this was not true in my case.

My Doctor, an Endocrinologist, actually raised my 120mg dose, to 150mg, so increased it 30mg, despite my low TSH. He said TSH in some patients, does not always accurately reflect some of the other thyroid lab levels.

In my case, this was due to my other endocrine glands, including my "pituitary" (regulates the thyroid), also operating at sub-clinically low levels, due to my also having CFS. Many medical sources state that CFS results in a "blunted HPA Axis" (hypothalamus-pituitary-adrenal axis).

CFS is more common in Thyroid Patients

He also said from all of my test results, including low adrenal hormones, a highly elevated Epstein-Barr Virus count, continually swollen lymph nodes in my throat etc..., that I have co-existing Chronic Fatigue Syndrome (CFS). I had already been told this by a chiropractic doctor, three years earlier. He also added that thyroid patients sometimes have multi-endocrine problems, when everything runs low in addition to the thyroid gland but is especially true if the patient also has CFS.

I asked him if CFS was found more commonly in thyroid disease patients and he said it was but is often not recognized by doctors and is sometimes attributed to thyroid treatment failure. This all amazed me because I had seen this Endocrinologist, 4 times previous and I had never asked him if he recognized CFS as a real syndrome/illness. He said he certainly does and he recognized it in me, without my having ever brought the subject of CFS up to him. Several years following this diagnosis of Hashimoto's and CFS, I have improved in many ways, especially when my thyroid is treated well, which reduces and helps control all symptoms significantly.

The Effect of Thyroid Flares on CFS Symptoms

I also asked my doctor if thyroid patients commonly have symptom flare-ups and he said any patient with autoimmune thyroid disease will have ups and downs with symptoms, due to antibody and inflammation levels fluctuating, which in turn causes thyroid hormones to also fluctuate slightly. I believe this is also an aspect in the symptom-levels of patients with co-morbid CFS and Fibromyalgia.

My doctor ordered follow up blood tests for me after two months on the increased thyroid med dose, asking for TSH, Free T-4 and Free T-3. My TSH was and is consistently below normal with blood retests but must be in my case due to my having co-morbid CFS. This keeps my thyroid hormone levels at mid-range and above, which most treated thyroid patients need to feel well.

Testing for Adrenal Fatigue

I haven't often shared about my struggles with the co-occurring CFS but have done relatively well with it much of the time and always remain positive about it. I do feel that thyroid patients with ongoing adrenal fatigue could possibly be experiencing a blunted HPA axis and co-morbid CFS.

If they suspect they have ongoing adrenal fatigue or CFS symptoms, they should ask for their adrenal hormone levels to be tested, preferably by multiple saliva samples over a 24 hour period, to better determine their cortisol rhythm.

Treating all Contributing Factors

My doctor did say that treating thyroid disease or any other underlying autoimmune condition is a major factor in helping control the symptoms of CFS and I know this has been true in my case. I also take adrenal support when needed that consists of a combination of vitamins, safe herbals and adrenal glandular supplement, which also helps control my symptoms of CFS and the adrenal fatigue that is a major feature of it.

{It is an incorrect view for medical sources to state that having thyroid disease, eliminates the possibility of having CFS because this is not true in some cases and in fact autoimmune diseases including thyroid ones, may be a trigger for causing co-existing CFS or Fibromyalgia. The U.S. NIH has changed on their stance in this regard and now states that CFS can be co morbid to endocrine illnesses.}

Improvements in my Symptoms

Since receiving treatment for these health disorders I have seen significant improvement in them. I do still experience flares of symptoms, if I venture outside of a diet restricting stimulants or if I do not keep my stress levels under control. It was my own experience that inspired me to research intensely on the subject of thyroid disease and how CFS and Fibromyalgia are often co-morbid to it. It is my belief that Chronic Fatigue Syndrome (CFS) has a type of adrenal exhaustion involved with it (one major aspect) and that adrenal fatigue can be a forerunner to it in some cases. The most well-established feature of CFS that you find in medical research (also Fibromyalgia), is "low cortisol levels" and I do not believe this is a coincidence but something that makes sense because the main purposes of cortisol is regulating stress and controlling inflammatory responses in the body. Two of the doctors I have been treated by since 2003, also diagnosed me with co-morbid CFS.

Healthy Adrenals Contribute to Healthy Immune Function

The adrenals when low functioning, cause more allergy, viral and illness responses to occur, due to the adrenals role in immune system function, being greatly diminished.

Common Diseases and Syndromes of Body Pain

Cortisol is also our body's naturalanti-inflammatory and so low levels give rise to joint & muscle pain and other inflammatory reactions in the body. All of these factors combined, contribute to the symptoms of adrenal fatigue, CFS and Fibromyalgia and can add to the symptom struggles of hypothyroid patients who have these co-morbid conditions.

CHAPTER SEVEN

More about CFS, Fibromyalgia and Low Cortisol

For more than twenty years, researchers studying Chronic Fatigue Syndrome (CFS) and Fibromyalgia Syndrome, have conducted studies in regard to adrenal function in patients with these syndromes and have concluded that patients are found to be experiencing "low adrenal function" as one of the features of these syndromes. This co-existing condition is also called "adrenal fatigue", "adrenal exhaustion" and "low adrenal reserve".

Through testing of a patient's adrenal hormones, it can be determined if that person has low-functioning adrenals. In addition to blood testing, saliva tests are also accurate for testing the "free levels" of the adrenal hormones, the main ones being DHEA and cortisol. A "24 hour urinary cortisol test" can also be done to test adrenal-cortisol levels.

Another major adrenal function blood test is also available, called the "ACTH Stimulation Test". This one is designed to confirm or rule out true "adrenal insufficiency" (full blown). Most CFS and Fibromyalgia patients do not have true, full blown adrenal insufficiency but a milder form of adrenal fatigue/exhaustion.

Medical Research - The Effect of CFS and FMS on Cortisol Levels

Research conclusions by major Medical Research groups, including the NIH, state that low cortical levels, are found to be a contributing factor in CFS/FMS, due to dysfunction of the HPA Axis (Hypothalamus-Pituitary-Adrenal Axis). It is my opinion because of this, that CFS/FMS has as one of its features, a form of adrenal fatigue, that does not meet the definition for true "adrenal insufficiency" and because of this, it cannot be medically treated the same. With full blown Adrenal Insufficiency, a much more serious condition, the low adrenal hormones must be replaced through steroid treatment (cortisone-steroid/hydrocortisone). With lesser forms of low adrenal function, such as adrenal fatigue, steroid treatment can possibly worsen the adrenal problem because the steroids may cause "adrenal suppression", which means the patient may have to take the steroids, the rest of their life because anything less than very short-term use of the steroids, can cause this suppression.

Triggers for CFS and FMS

Some of the other things Medical Researchers have studied in regard to CFS and Fibromyalgia, is the fact that these syndromes can have different triggers for different patients.

Common Diseases and Syndromes of Body Pain

For many, it is an underlying viral, autoimmune, bacterial etc..., type infection in the body, that causes chronic activation of the immune system and over time, this uses up some of the adrenal reserves because the adrenals have a major role in releasing cortisol, the body's natural anti-inflammatory, attempting to ward off inflammation.

Cortisol (also called "cortical"), is also the "stress hormone", that helps the body to deal with stresses of all kinds, without it, even the smallest stressor would cause shock and death (adrenal crises). It, along with adrenaline, are "fight or flight" hormones and help protect the body from the effects of stress, from minor emotional stress, to major ones, such as a car accident or serious disease.

Diminished Tolerance to Stressors

This in my opinion is why persons with CFS/FMS have such low tolerance for stressors both emotional and physical. With low adrenal function, even mild emotional and physical stresses result in major fatigue, couple this with the immune system dysfunction that CFS/FMS patients also have and you have syndromes with serious symptoms! It may be that the immune deficiency found in both CFS and Fibromyalgia is also a type of burn-out of that system, due to constant, ongoing activation of it, that the body eventually loses the ability to continue.

Common Diseases and Syndromes of Body Pain

As with all other opinions about CFS and Fibromyalgia, we have to consider all of the above, as some of the many theories that are out there however, I feel the evidence of low adrenal function in CFS and Fibromyalgia is overwhelming. What I have described, is what I feel connects these syndromes to a form of adrenal fatigue.

Stress is a known trigger for adrenal fatigue and related syndromes, such as Chronic Fatigue Syndrome and Fibromyalgia and it can also bring an autoimmune disease to the surface, that is in the body but hasn't fully manifested and thyroid diseases are some of the more common ones that are triggered by stress, especially Grave's Disease/hyperthyroidism.

PTSD (Post Traumatic stress Disorder) is also a chronic stress caused syndrome as mentioned previously but is also classified as an anxiety disorder.

Chronic Stressors – A Precursor to Stress Related Syndromes

I personally went through an extreme, chronic time of stress and my thyroid disease, called "Hashimoto's Thyroiditis" and adrenal fatigue manifested because of it. I was untreated for several months and the result was an added severe flare-up I experienced, that I know for a fact triggered an even more severe CFS form of adrenal fatigue in me (Chronic Fatigue syndrome).

Common Diseases and Syndromes of Body Pain

I initially developed severe hives and a strange viral type illness that left me with the CFS. After this, the lymph nodes in my neck remained swollen to this day and I have severe chemical sensitivities.

My belief is that CFS is an altered HPA Axis ("blunted"), plus altered immune function syndrome combined, so I do try to tell people to get their adrenal hormones and all other hormones checked as well, including the sex hormones because it is my belief that hormonal imbalances over time, can possibly result in CFS and Fibromyalgia type illnesses.

Some who read my articles or have read my posts on forums, may wonder why I have the passion I do for the adrenal subjects and it is because it is my belief that adrenal fatigue can contribute to the development of CFS and/or FMS type syndromes, when not taken seriously and investigated/treated if a patient has it.

Working Toward Recovery

Things that speed recovery for CFS include:

• treating the adrenal fatigue
• getting a lot of sleep and rest
• a healthy diet
• exercising to tolerance ...

Common Diseases and Syndromes of Body Pain

...

• making sure other diseases a patient might have are treated properly

Under-treatment of a thyroid disorder for example, can serve as a trigger for CFS flare-ups and may actually be a trigger for the syndrome itself according to some medical sources.

For many with CFS, chronic stress was a trigger for the onset of the syndrome.

CHAPTER EIGHT

The Connection of Epstein-Barr Virus to CFS and Fibromyalgia

The EBV (Epstein-Barr Virus), which causes Mononucleosis initially in some patients can afterward, remain in a persons body for life. This virus is suspected of having a strong connection to CFS.

While most people with EBV in their system (estimates are 80 to 95% of the population), only have antibody titers to the virus, that are just barely positive, like a "5", a "10", "20" above normal, etc..., others actually have flare-ups of this virus, probably due to a compromised immune system (immune deficiency) that causes really high counts/titers of the virus to increase in their bodies over time.

Many in the medical field are of the opinion that EBV is a background virus like many others in the herpes virus-family, that can flare-up like cold sores can (also a herpes virus). When flare-ups happen, they believe it causes or at least contributes to symptoms of CFS.

In my case, my EBV count was "218" with normal range being <20, so mine was more than ten times the normal cut off range.

Common Diseases and Syndromes of Body Pain

EBV – An Indicator of Immune Function

Some Doctors believe the EBV test means nothing, unless actually being used to test for Mononucleosis but there has to be a reason some patient's EBV counts elevate so highly. Both MDs I now go to, believe that EBV can flare-up in some patients who have high titers of it. Many sources also state that adrenal fatigue is a major feature of this because the adrenals are the major moderators of our immune system.

While EBV may not be the actual root cause of CFS, it has been shown to be an indicator of immune dysfunction in studies that have been conducted. In my opinion, it is just one of many factors that can contribute to the symptoms of CFS. In addition to EBV, other herpes-family viruses suspected in the cause of CFS and Fibromyalgia include the human herpes virus 6 (HHV-6), Cytomegalovirus (also a herpes virus) and Coxsackie viruses B1 and B4.

CHAPTER NINE

More on Symptoms and Diagnosis of Fibromyalgia

Widespead and Chronic Muscle Pain

Fibromyalgia is a syndrome of widespread body pain and fatigue. There are signs and symptoms that can help to identify and diagnose Fibromyalgia.

People with Fibromyalgia syndrome (FMS) will find that they experience widespread and severe body pain that is chronic (ongoing). The pain will affect the muscles and joints but will also produce "tender points." These are places on the body that experience pain when pressure is applied to them, where muscles are attached to bones, at the joints. Some in the medical community vary in their opinions as to whether FMS is a rheumatic condition or strictly a pain syndrome. Others believe it is a combination of both.

Published Diagnostic Criteria

In addition to also being recognized as an inflammatory disorder, some research studies have also found that FMS may be an autoimmune-related disorder. Some medical research groups have also found that FMS and Chronic Fatigue Syndrome (CFS) have 75% crossover symptom similarities as mentioned previously.

Common Diseases and Syndromes of Body Pain

Some published diagnostic studies have suggested that Fibromyalgia is better determined when a person experiencing FMS symptoms is found to have at least 11 of the 18 possible tender points that can occur throughout the body. These are areas where pain will occur upon applying mild pressure to them, using a fingertip.

The areas on the body where these tender points may occur include the following:
• the hips
• the knees
• the back of the head near the base of the neck
• upper areas of the chest
• the upper back in the cervical spine area
• the elbows
• the shoulders

Fatigue and Sleep Disturbances

Fatigue is another major symptom of FMS and it is sometimes exacerbated by sleep disturbances that can also occur. The fatigue is often relentless and proper sleep and rest does little to alleviate it completely. Normal circadian sleep rhythms (cycles) that are supposed to occur become abnormal in Fibromyalgia patients, which results in daytime sleepiness and feeling more awake during nighttime hours.

Common Diseases and Syndromes of Body Pain

Medical research, including that conducted by the National Institutes of Health (U.S.-NIH), suggests that abnormal functioning of the adrenal glands is one possible cause of the disrupted sleep patterns, due to the adrenal hormone "cortisol" not being properly regulated by the adrenal glands in people who have Fibromyalgia.

Digestive Disturbances and IBS

FMS patients may complain of severe indigestion, heartburn and acid reflux with FMS but may also experience alternating spells of constipation and diarrhea. This may indicate that they are also suffering from Irritable Bowel Syndrome (IBS). Frequent gastritis and bloating may also manifest as part of the digestive problems that can occur with Fibromyalgia.

Headaches and Sensory Disturbances

Many people with Fibromyalgia experience frequent headaches and these may have a neurological aspect to them that they have not experienced previously. The headaches may sometimes have an unusual pattern to them or will affect the person's senses as they occur (i.e. eyesight, sense of smell, taste and hearing). These sensory changes can occur with headaches or may also occur without them.

These may include heightened and/or loss of sensitivity to the following:

- light
- noises
- flavors
- odors
- sense of touch

Emotional and Mental Symptoms

People with FMS may also experience symptoms of anxiety and depression and a change in mental functioning. These emotional symptoms may alternate between those of anxiety and depression or the patient may experience mostly one of these mood problems. A person with Fibromyalgia may experience anxiety symptoms as an increase in chronic worry and episodes of fear, including the possibility of panic attacks. The depression may be perceived by them as a profound sadness, an emptiness or hopelessness.

This demonstrates the importance in monitoring Fibromyalgia patients for any signs of worsening emotional symptoms, which may require treatment as a separate issue, in addition to treatments that are needed for rheumatic symptoms (muscle pain).

Mental functioning may also become diminished in Fibromyalgia patients. They may have difficulty concentrating and will experience what is often referred to as "brain fog," a term to describe mental dullness or an inability to focus with the same sharpness they had previous to their illness. Short-term memory loss is also experience in some FMS patients.

See Your Doctor

People who experience the symptoms described in the subheadings above need to see a qualified, licensed medial physician in order to confirm a diagnosis of Fibromyalgia or other conditions with similar symptoms. Patients receiving a diagnosis of FMS can move forward with appropriate treatment, which can help to control symptoms or diminish them significantly and return them to an improved quality of life.

CHAPTER TEN

More on the Suspected Causes of CFS

Triggers for Chronic Fatigue Syndrome

Decades of medical research on Chronic Fatigue Syndrome has revealed a number of abnormalities in patients with the syndrome. One definitive cause has yet to be found.

Chronic Fatigue Syndrome (CFS) is a complicated and sometimes mysterious illness. Medical research studies have been ongoing for many years in attempts to find a definitive cause for the illness. Medical groups studying CFS have instead found a number of aspects of the syndrome that are clearly present but each may play a role or be one of the many factors of CFS rather than its definitive cause.

Post Viral Illness

A number of viruses studied in relation to CFS have been found to be present in significant titers (lab result measurements) in people suffering the syndrome. Among the viruses suspected of being possible causes or triggers for CFS, are enteroviruses and retroviruses.

These include the Epstein-Barr Virus (EBV) that is usually contracted during childhood and carried throughout one's lifetime, human herpesvirus 6 and the Cytomegalovirus. Candida albican overgrowth (fungal/yeast infection), although not in the virus category has also been suspected as a possible cause or trigger for CFS.

Some of these viruses, including EBV cause no symptoms in most people when contracted (can potentially cause mononucleosis) but will increase in the number of titers found in the blood when the virus replicates. It has been proposed as a possibility that the increased replication of viruses may occur when the immune system is not functioning well in suppressing their ability to replicate or reactivate. Reactivation would mean that a virus resurges at times, causing repeated illness in the infected person who has not fully developed immunity to it.

Imbalance in the Involuntary Nervous System

In other studies of CFS patients, they have been found to be experiencing dysfunction in their involuntary nervous systems (INS), also referred to as "autonomic failure" and "dysautonomia".

The INS is responsible for regulating blood pressure with changes in physical activity and changes in positions of the body (i.e. sitting, standing and lying flat).

Common Diseases and Syndromes of Body Pain

It also regulates all other involuntary bodily functions, including respiration, digestion, kidney function, liver function, etc... and increases these functions when needed (sympathetic response) or decreases them (parasympathetic response).

An imbalance in this system will cause these functions to be inadequate at times and over-responsive at other times. If for example, physical activity is increased and blood pressure needs to rise but fails to do so, this can result in bodily fatigue due to a lack of needed blood flow to the muscles and organs of the body. If bodily functions need to decrease at times of rest or when sleep is needed but remain highly activated this will result in fatigue as well.

Dysfunction of the Immune System

Other, conclusions resulting from medical studies of CFS causes, has found that patients with the syndrome are experiencing a dysfunction of the immune system. The immunity or what might be referred to as "resistance" to viruses and allergens is greatly diminished in CFS patients. This means that the body is more susceptible to viruses and allergens and recovers more slowly from exposure and infections to them, than are people with healthy immune systems.

Infections of these types can cause a mild systemic (system-wide) inflammation in the body and cause the person experiencing them, to feel as if they are experiencing perpetual flu-like symptoms or a continual low-grade fever.

Chronic Stress

CFS patients often report in medical study questionnaires that they experienced severe, prolonged or traumatic stress, just before the onset of their CFS symptoms. Stress is responded-to by the part of the endocrine system called the "HPA Axis", standing for the Hypothalamus-Pituitary-Adrenal gland system. When chronic stress is experienced, this system is hyper-active and over time, becomes "blunted", meaning it becomes fatigued or diminished in its ability to run at overdrive. This causes slower release of the hormones that come from these endocrine glands that work in sync (full-circle) to supply the body with stress coping abilities.

The end result of the hypothalamus stimulating the pituitary gland, which then in-turn stimulates the adrenal glands, is the release of the stress hormone "cortisol". When this system becomes blunted after extended hyperactivity, cortisol levels begin to fall or what is sometimes referred to as "hypocortisolemia" or "hypoadrenia". Some sources recognizing this mild form of adrenal dysfunction refer to it as "Adrenal Fatigue".

Common Diseases and Syndromes of Body Pain

CHAPTER ELEVEN

Treatments for CFS and Fibromyalgia

There have been no cures found for either of these syndromes and so the treatments are to reduce the symptoms of them. Some patients do see complete recovery but there is no solid medically confirmed proof that treatment of the symptoms is what brought recovery in these cases.

Since the symptoms of these two syndromes crossover significantly, let me first mention the specific treatment for Fibromyalgia patients who have significantly severe muscle and joint pain. Following that, I will list the treatments that are commonly administered for both syndromes.

Fibromyalgia patients are often given medications to control the pain in their muscles and joints. Some are also given anti-inflammatory drugs, to reduce inflammation that can also occur and that can contribute to the pain symptoms. These include over-the-counter and prescription pain and anti-inflammatory medications and corticosteroids (hydrocortisone), also called glucocorticoids.

Treatments that are commonly administered for both syndromes include correction of hormonal, vitamin, mineral and nutritional deficiencies of any kind, found through thorough blood lab testing. Hormones that may be low in these syndromes include:

• thyroid

• adrenal

• sex

Correction of these can significantly improve symptoms, as can correction of any other important body elements (i.e. minerals and nutrients) that may be found to be low.

Some patients see improvement in both emotional and physical symptoms when administered SSRI antidepressants. A therapy called "Cognitive Behavioral Therapy" (CBT) can also be successful in relieving symptoms in some patients, as well as giving them skills for coping with their illness.

Since Adrenal Fatigue (low cortisol) is a major feature of these syndromes, the following treatment recommended for this stress-related aspect, can also improve symptoms significantly.

Common Diseases and Syndromes of Body Pain

Get more Sleep, Rest and Relaxation

In today's fast-paced society, a busy schedule can leave little time for adequate sleep, rest and relaxation. This lack of rest can heighten your stress level and place too much demand on the adrenal glands. Like any organ or gland of the body, the adrenals need time to rest in order to rebuild their reserves and abilities to function at optimal level. The job of these glands is to supply the body with adequate levels of adrenal hormones, but they can only do this if the body in general is allowed to rest and relax for sufficient periods of time.

Medical sources state that most people need a minimum of eight hours of sleep per night in order to function at their best level during the daytime and in order for the cells of the body to have adequate time to repair and restore from normal use of the body.

Our everyday routines also place a degree of stress upon our minds and emotions. While sleep is very important to get in adequate amounts, so is simple rest and relaxation in general. If you don't allow for leisure time and time to simply sit or lie down and rest on occasion, you will not be allowing your body and mind to unwind from the stressors of everyday duties and this leads to that feeling of being "stressed out" by the end of the day or even before the end of the day.

People with full time jobs are many times actually required by their employers to provide them two breaks per day, to take a short rest of usually 20 minutes per break. This is due to studies that indicate even short rest periods help workers rejuvenate their energies, in order to continue and complete their work days more efficiently. Rest, sleep and relaxation are also necessary to prevent or recover from adrenal fatigue.

Reduce your Stress Levels

No one living in the world today can escape or be immune to stress. Stress is a fact of life; our goal is to work on reducing its effects and learn coping skills, so that we find ways to eliminate as much of it as we possibly can. The adrenal glands help us to cope with and to recover from stress by providing the body with adequate levels of the stress hormone "cortisol".

This hormone is also considered to be a "fight or flight" hormone, just like adrenaline. But while adrenaline is the more short term energizing hormone needed at times of danger (to escape or fight a situation or enemy), cortisol is the long term fight or flight hormone, giving us the needed flow of energy, throughout the day, to perform our normal tasks.

Common Diseases and Syndromes of Body Pain

Relentless and ongoing stress can eventually use up the reserves of this hormone faster than the adrenals are able to supply it, unless we allow ourselves time to recuperate from stress. Only then can the adrenals rebuild the reserves of this very important stress hormone and the others it also supplies to the body. Stress can be reduced simply by resting and giving ourselves time during each day to unwind for a few minutes at a time.

It is also important not to get uptight throughout the day over small problems that arise. We should learn to not take the smaller problems as seriously, because there are potentially too many of them that can arise and this will keep our stress levels peaked too often or for extended periods.

In addition to taking "timeouts" to unwind during the day, we can also involve ourselves in hobbies or leisure activities that give us pleasure during our times away from work, further helping us to relax and unwind. Involving yourself in enjoyable activities can provide you with much needed enjoyment-of-life that helps you relieve stress and feel more refreshed when the time for work returns.

Common Diseases and Syndromes of Body Pain

Take Supplements that help Strengthen the Adrenals

There are many supplements that can be taken to help keep the body and adrenal glands healthy and strengthened so they can handle the everyday stress life brings upon all of us. A really good multi-vitamin is always a great idea and there are many good ones out there to choose from. Some major vitamin companies actually make vitamins called "stress formulas" or "stress tabs" and these contain the vitamins and minerals that help the body cope with and recover from stress.

Additional vitamin supplements in particular that are very helpful to the adrenal glands include "B" vitamins – in particular, B-12, B-5 and B-6. Vitamin "C" is also an important vitamin for healthy adrenal function. Minerals that can help with adrenal function include zinc and magnesium. There are also adrenal herbal formulas that contain helpful supplements, but these should be researched carefully by anyone who is considering taking them and also discussed with your doctor before taking them. Purchase supplements only from reliable, reputable companies.

Other natural supplements to be taken after observing these precautions include "adrenal glandular" (usually beef source), "licorice root extract" (helps adrenals produce more cortisol) and DHEA (over-the-counter adrenal hormone).

Common Diseases and Syndromes of Body Pain

Some Adrenal Fatigue sufferers also report improvement using herbal and other energy supplements such as Ashwagandha, Ginseng, Ribrose and Co-Q10.

All of these supplements can potentially be helpful, but everyone is unique; some supplements work better for some than others and sometimes it simply takes a trial of several of these to find the one that eventually helps the most. Also make sure you thoroughly research any supplements you plan to take, discuss them with your doctor and only take the manufacture's recommended dose or that set by your doctor.

Incorporate Regular Exercise into your Health Regimen

Exercise is important in strengthening the body in general. Regular exercise also results in strengthened adrenal glands. Doctors know that exercise helps the hormones in our bodies to do their jobs better because it helps to circulate and metabolize them better. Cortisol, the stress hormone produced by the adrenals, also helps to regulate our glucose (blood sugar) and is one reason exercise helps in this process.

When you begin an exercise routine, it is important that you do so at the pace your body can tolerate. You do not want to overdo on exercise; too much exercise will not increase the benefit from it faster, but can actually have an adverse effect.

This is especially true of people who are already experiencing adrenal fatigue. They can have reduced tolerance for exercise and if they do not pace themselves, they can worsen the adrenal fatigue rather than helping resolve it.

Walking is one of the best exercises to start out with, and a good everyday exercise for anyone. Some who start with walking can eventually progress to jogging, if that's what they chose and they are healthy enough to do so. If you prefer walking as your exercise, many sources state that walking 15 to 20 minutes at least three times a week will provide a healthy benefit, and five times or more per week increases that benefit.

See a licensed professional - medical practitioner when seeking the diagnosis and treatment of Chronic Fatigue Syndrome or Fibromyalgia.

(END-SECTION TWO)

Common Diseases and Syndromes of Body Pain

SECTION THREE:

Neuropathy and Myopathy in Treated Thyroid Disease

Hypothyroid and Hyperthyroid Nerve Pain and Muscle Weakness

TABLE OF CONTENTS:

INTRODUCTION:

Thyroid disease patients can experience a number of different complications as a result of their hypothyroid (underactive thyroid) or hyperthyroid (overactive thyroid) conditions. Two of these complications are nerve pain and dysfunction, referred to as "peripheral neuropathy" and muscle weakness with possible atrophy (shrinkage of muscles), referred to as "thyroid myopathy".

In some cases, these two problems that are co-morbid to thyroid disorders can coexist, so that they are occurring at the same time and this may be referred to as "neuromuscular disease". This is a symptom-aspect that has less information available on it via online medical search, than do the more common thyroid-related problems, such as weight gain, joint pain and fatigue.

Within the chapters of this book, that follow, I hope to present to the reader, a general understanding of these often debilitating and potentially very serious manifestations of thyroid disease, affecting the nerves and muscles of the body, including the treatments available for them. I present this information to you as a fellow hypothyroid patient with autoimmune thyroiditis and co-morbid peripheral neuropathy and myopathy, which inspired me to search and research the information contained in the chapters.

Common Diseases and Syndromes of Body Pain

CHAPTER ONE

What Components of Thyroid Disease causes Neuropathy and/or Myopathy?

After reading much of the medical research that is available regarding peripheral neuropathy and myopathy that results from thyroid disease, I have come to the conclusion that these problems can potentially result from the autoimmune aspect of thyroid disease or from the metabolic aspect of it or as a result of both these components, simultaneously.

While myopathy is simply a term for muscle weakness that can include atrophy (muscle wasting), peripheral neuropathy is a term that includes sensory symptoms (i.e. burning, tingling and numbness), motor symptoms (i.e. muscle weakness and difficulty controlling movements in them) and autonomic symptoms (i.e. changes in involuntary body functions, such as digestion, sweating, cardiopulmonary and other organ functions).

In some patients with nerve pain, only one limb or area of their body is affected (mono-neuropathy), while others see many areas of the body affected simultaneously (poly-neuropathy).

Autoimmune Hypothyroidism

The autoimmune aspect of thyroid disease that can be involved in the previously-described symptoms and others is the disease process that results in hormone imbalances of either the underactive or overactive thyroid types. The underactive type, also referred to as "hypothyroidism", is often the result of auto-antibodies from the immune system, that mistakenly attack the thyroid gland, which is referred to as autoimmune thyroiditis.

The types of hypothyroid autoimmunity are somewhat varied but the most common type in industrialized countries is "Hashimoto's disease", also referred to as "chronic lymphocytic thyroiditis". This common form of thyroiditis, results from the creation of auto-antibodies, from the immune system, that attack key thyroid proteins that are responsible for the manufacture of thyroid hormones, from iodine that enters the body via the diet.

These two key proteins are the "thyroid Peroxidase" and the "thyroglobulin" and when these are attacked and destroyed by auto-antibodies, they are referred to as the "anti-thyroidperoxidase" and "anti-thyroglobulin" antibodies (abbreviated on blood lab tests as "Anti-TPO" and anti-TG").

Common Diseases and Syndromes of Body Pain

These eventually cause enough damage and destruction to the thyroid gland as to cause it to manufacture abnormally low levels of thyroid hormone, which reduces the speed of metabolism in the body. The purpose of these hormones is to regulate a proper level of metabolism -- the production of energy that results from things consumed into the body (i.e. food, water and oxygen).

Autoimmune Hyperthyroidism

In the case of autoimmune overactive thyroid gland disease, also referred to as "Graves' disease", the type of auto-antibodies that cause the opposite effect of abnormally high thyroid antibodies in the body, are called "thyroid stimulating immunoglobulin" (abbreviated "TSI"). These are sent from the immune system and attach to key proteins in the thyroid gland, causing them to become overly-stimulated in producing thyroid hormone from iodine.

Some medical sources state that the TSI antibody mimics the effects of a naturally occurring hormone sent from the pituitary brain-gland, called "thyroid stimulating hormone" (abbreviated "TSH"). The pituitary gland fluctuates in the level of this necessary hormone that it sends to the thyroid gland, to properly regulate the amount of thyroid hormones manufactured and dispersed throughout all the cells of the body.

Common Diseases and Syndromes of Body Pain

It does-so, by sensing how much of these hormones the body needs at any given time, the main ones being the "T4" (containing 4 iodine molecules) and the "T3" (containing 3 iodine molecules). It is a very sensitive system that adjusts to physical activity levels and other factors that require changes in bodily metabolism but it becomes disrupted when the thyroid gland is being attacked by either hypothyroid or hyperthyroid causing antibodies.

Autoimmunity of any kind is a strange thing. With autoimmune diseases, the body begins to attack itself for reasons that we simply have no understanding of at this stage; this despite there being significant numbers of medical research studies on the subject that have been published by medical groups for decades. For some reason, the immune system will begin to attack natural, normal tissues in the body, as if they are something that presents a danger to the rest of the body. These specially-created antibodies are usually sent-out to destroy viruses and bacteria or to control allergens that might enter the body via airborne particles that are breathed-in or that are consumed in food or water. When a part of the body that does not present a threat to us is attacked by this autoimmune response, apart from these obvious reasons, it is a mystery to medical doctors and researchers who diagnose and study diseases of autoimmunity.

Common Diseases and Syndromes of Body Pain

Bodily Metabolism Depends on Thyroid Hormones

Since both the muscles and nerves are highly dependent upon a normal metabolism to operate correctly, they can become negatively hindered and possibly damaged by thyroid hormone imbalances that are severe or when treatment is delayed for them.

My belief after corresponding with literally 100s of fellow-thyroid patients since the year 2003 is that some patients experience problems with neuropathy and/or myopathy, even after receiving adequate or optimal thyroid treatment and I am in-fact one of them.

The "metabolic aspect" of thyroid disease previously described which causes either a slowed hypothyroid metabolism or a sped-up hyperthyroid metabolism can be a factor that causes development of neuropathy and myopathy as well. This is true even if it is secondarily-caused, rather than being a problem within the thyroid gland itself.

Secondary causes of thyroid dysfunction result from other problems within the body, that affect thyroid hormone production but that still affect bodily metabolism as a result, due to an imbalance in the hormones.

If the pituitary gland for example, becomes disrupted due to a tumor that develops within it, this can cause it to either slow-down or speed-up the dispersing of TSH to the thyroid gland. This is referred to as "central hypothyroidism" and "central hyperthyroidism", meaning there is a problem occurring in the brain-center from which proper thyroid regulation normally originates. In females, tumors on the ovaries can be a secondary cause of an overactive thyroid gland as well.

Small tumors within the thyroid gland itself, called "hot nodules" which would actually be a "primary cause" of hyperthyroidism but that can occur without thyroid autoimmunity being present, can also develop. A long-term, uncorrected abnormal increase or decrease in metabolism due to thyroid hormone imbalances can become detrimental to the body.

Symptoms of Thyroid Hormone Disorders

When <u>hypothyroidism</u> occurs due to any cause, the resulting symptoms can include the following.

• Muscle and joint aches
• Nerve pain in the extremities

• Feeling cold in warm temperatures

• Dry skin and brittle fingernails ...

Common Diseases and Syndromes of Body Pain

...

• Hair that has become brittle and breaks off or falls out

• Thinning of the eyebrows and loss of the outer 1/3 portion of them

• Unexplained weight gain with no diet change

• Constipation

• Slowed heart rate and breathing

• Depression

• Physical tiredness/fatigue
• Myxedema (fluid retention-tissue swelling)

• Feeling a fullness or tightness in the throat (goiter)

When hyperthyroidism occurs due to any cause, the resulting symptoms can include the following.

• Muscle and joint aches aches (possible muscle atrophy)
• Nerve pain in the extremities
• Rapid heart rate
• Hyperventilation
• Hypertension
• Sweating
• Inability to sleep
• Nervousness and anxiety
• Diarrhea ...

Common Diseases and Syndromes of Body Pain

...
• Excessive energy followed by fatigue
• Hair loss
• Weight loss
• Osteoporosis (bone loss)
• Myxedema
• Swelling of the thyroid gland (goiter)

In many cases the "myxedema" symptom, shown in both lists, is directly related to nerve pain in the body due to fluid-retention causing excessive pressure on the nerves. When either of these thyroid hormone imbalances has been diagnosed, treatment for them will begin. In the chapter that follows, diagnoses methods and treatments will be discussed.

CHAPTER TWO

Treatments for Hypothyroid and Hyperthyroid Hormone Imbalances

For both hypothyroid and hyperthyroid disorders, blood lab testing is often the type of diagnostic method that first detects them. A panel is often ordered when symptoms indicate a thyroid hormone imbalance is present and it will often consist of the T4, T3 and TSH levels.

If additional labs are ordered, these will usually be imaging tests, such as radioactive iodine uptake scans, thyroid ultrasound, MRI, CAT scans and occasionally, a fine-needle tissue biopsy is extracted from the thyroid gland for analysis.

The Sensitivity of TSH Blood Testing

If a thyroid condition is not suspected and a patient is simply having a battery of tests ordered for a routine medical evaluation, the only test that might be included to evaluate thyroid function will be the TSH. This test is often the most sensitive for detecting a lowering or increasing T4 and/or T3 level.

The reason for this being, that TSH is increased to abnormally high levels, to maintain proper thyroid hormone levels when they are decreased even slightly, due to a diseased thyroid gland or due to a secondary cause resulting in hypothyroidism.

If the gland has begun to produce too-much thyroid hormone due to primary or secondary hyperthyroidism the opposite will occur and the TSH will begin to drop to below-normal levels, even early into the thyroid over-activity. During this process, the pituitary gland may be able to correct the T4 and T3 for a period of time but it struggles to do so and eventually the thyroid hormones also become imbalanced, as the TSH fails to maintain them at normal values.

Many patients' thyroid disorders first manifest with an abnormal TSH and the T4 and T3 will remain temporarily-normal at this juncture. This is referred-to as "subclinical thyroid disorder" and for many patients; their condition will stay at a subclinical stage for months or even years.

If a patient experiences symptoms of either overactive or underactive thyroid glands, even when only the TSH is abnormal, some doctors will begin treatment at this stage. If symptoms are not present with an abnormal TSH level, a doctor might instead retest the patients' blood level of TSH, every few months to see if the disorder is progressing to an overt level (full blown).

Common Diseases and Syndromes of Body Pain

When Do Doctors Start Treatment for Thyroid Disorders?

Different thyroid-specializing doctors use a different standard for determining when to treat developing hypothyroid and hyperthyroid disorders. Some doctors will treat hypothyroid patients whose TSH is elevated but whose T4 and T3 levels are normal, as long as TSH reaches a level of at-least "10.0" or higher (the highest normal value at labs, currently averages about "5.0").

Some doctors will also treat hypothyroid patients if both the TSH is elevated and the T4 or T3 are below normal on blood test results. Yet other doctors factor-in the presence or absence of symptoms, as previously mentioned.

The same type logic is used by some doctors in regard to hyperthyroid conditions as well but in this case, the TSH lowest normal value averages approximately "0.3" at testing labs, currently. If a hyperthyroid patient has indications of an overactive metabolism (symptoms), with a below-normal TSH but their T4 and T3 remain within normal values, the doctor may opt to start them on treatment as well and most doctors will certainly do-so if both TSH is abnormally low and the T4 and/or T3 are abnormally high.

Types of Thyroid Disease Treatments

Hypothyroidism treatment is relatively simple compared to treatments for hyperthyroidism and consists of simply supplementing the hypothyroid patient with a daily dose of T4 or combination T4 and T3 hormone replacement medication. The prescribed dose will correct the low thyroid hormone levels over time but this might take a process of several months, with the dose starting at a minimal level and being titrated upward (adjusted by gradual increases), until the patients' TSH, T4 and T3 levels return to adequate or optimal normal values. This is determined via repeat blood testing, every few weeks or months.

Hyperthyroidism treatments are slightly more complicated and varied, depending on the cause of the overactive thyroid gland and the severity of it. In some cases, a patient will only require the prescribing of an "anti-thyroid drug", which slows the production of thyroid hormones, returning thyroid function to a normal level.

Other patients might need a beta-blocker medication prescribed, which will correct hypertension and tachycardia (rapid heart rate) if these are present and if an anti-thyroid drug alone does not correct them. A combination of both type drugs can in some cases, correct the hyperthyroidism symptoms more adequately.

Some hyperthyroid patients need corrective surgeries, to move part or all of their thyroid glands (partial or total thyroidectomy) or they will be referred for radioactive iodine ablation of the gland.

This latter mentioned procedure, abbreviated "RAI" is performed by a qualified doctor who administers a dose of radioactive iodine to a patient, which is immediately absorbed by the gland and causes destruction of all tissues within it, so that it is basically dissolved/removed from the body within several weeks following the treatment.

Many doctors are now seeing more value in surgical removal because this often assures that the diseased thyroid tissue is fully removed. Thyroidectomy also becomes necessary in cases of thyroid cancer or when hot nodules are present but in the case of non-malignant nodules, only partial removal may become necessary.

Once thyroid removal of either type has been completed, the patient will require thyroid hormone replacement therapy, similar to that of hypothyroid patients, due to their thyroid glands not being fully present or not present at all, to supply thyroid hormone for proper bodily metabolism.

Is Prescribed Thyroid Hormone Always Adequate?

While these treatments correct thyroid hormone imbalances, some patients may still go on to see progression of neuropathy or myopathy symptoms. As stated earlier, my belief is that the "autoimmune" aspect of thyroid diseases may be responsible for this or it is also possible that supplemented thyroid hormones do not nourish the body and its metabolism as well as do naturally-occurring thyroid hormones.

This second possibility is certainly a theory at this point however, even the pharmaceutical companies who manufacture synthetic and natural brands of prescribed thyroid hormones, claim that certain competing brands do not as adequately resolve the complications of hypothyroid conditions.

Inadequacies in some manufactured hormones have actually resulted in the FDA requiring recalls of certain types, after dosage-inconsistencies were found in them (pharmacies required to take the product off-sale). Even the major brand manufacturers have been affected by these recalls in past years.

CHAPTER THREE

Why Thyroid Treatments may not Resolve Neuropathy and Myopathy Symptoms

There are a number of reasons why thyroid disease treatments might not fully resolve cases of peripheral neuropathy or thyroid myopathy. As mentioned in the previous chapter, one reason could be that thyroid hormones coming into the body from the outside (prescribed), rather than from the thyroid gland, naturally, may be less adequate.

As also previously mentioned, thyroid hormone replacement is not just required by hypothyroid patients but also by hyperthyroid patients who have had thyroidectomies or radioactive iodine ablations performed on them.

Undertreated Hypothyroid Patients

Some doctors, who are less-qualified to administer thyroid hormone replacement therapy, may also have a tendency to under-treat some patients. This can be due to the concern some doctors have for inducing thyrotoxicity (over-treatment causing hyperthyroidism) and as a result, they are reluctant to optimize treatment for patients to prevent the risk of inducing hyperthyroid symptoms.

Common Diseases and Syndromes of Body Pain

Under-treated patients carry the risk of complications from what amounts to being kept in a subclinical hypothyroid state by their doctors, including those affecting nerves and muscles.

Once Damage has been Done

I also believe that it's entirely possible that once nerve or muscle damage has occurred in thyroid patients, whether from hyperthyroid or hypothyroid conditions, the treatments they receive may not stop progression of further damage or the preceding damage is not fully reversible.

Medical sources that inform the public about "Thyroid Myopathy", state that the disease can be progressive, similar to types of muscular dystrophy and it becomes a disease entity of itself. Once this occurs, treatments are designed to address symptoms and to comfort patients as much as possible, rather than to reverse the disease process, if it has been established that it is irreversible.

Sensory, Autonomic and Motor Nerves

This same applies to some cases of peripheral neuropathy (PN), which once damaging the nerves, continues to cause sensory symptoms, such as burning, tingling and stabbing pains to the extremities via the "sensory nerves".

Common Diseases and Syndromes of Body Pain

This can progress to the trunk of the body and to the nerves that regulate involuntary organ functions as well (autonomic neuropathy).

If the "motor nerves" are also affected by a case of PN (those that affect muscle strength and movement), this may in some cases be placed into the category of a neuromuscular disease. This is not common and is more likely to occur in thyroid patients with other autoimmune diseases (i.e. Lupus, Rheumatoid Arthritis, Celiac disease and Sjogren 's syndrome) and in those with co-morbid diabetes than in those with thyroid disease only.

In my personal case however, I have had other autoimmune diseases and diabetes ruled-out repeatedly but I continue to experience neuropathy and myopathy symptoms, even after more than eight years of hypothyroid treatment, that has been optimized best-possible.

Research Regarding Neuropathy and Myopathy in Treated Thyroid Patients

Following are quotes from the U.S. National Institutes of Health (PubMed), regarding unresolved neuropathy and myopathy in treated hypothyroid patients, from five different research studies. ...

1.**Pain and small-fiber neuropathy in patients with hypothyroidism** (U.S. National Library of Medicine - PubMed) ---

"Conclusions: Some patients treated for hypothyroidism have symptoms and findings compatible with small-fiber neuropathy or "hyper phenomena" indicating central sensitization. ...of Eighteen patients...Eight were classified as having large fiber neuropathy..."

2.**Hypothyroidism and polyneuropathy.** (U.S. National Library of Medicine - PubMed) ---

"Using standard electrophysiological criteria, a definite diagnosis of polyneuropathy was made in 28 cases (72%). The commonest sites of abnormal nerve conduction were the sensory nerves, especially the sural nerve."

3.**Hypothyroid neuropathy and myopathy: clinical and electrodiagnostic longitudinal findings.** (U.S. National Library of Medicine - PubMed) ---

"This case shows that thyroid hormone replacement eliminates the neuropathic manifestations of severe hypothyroidism. In contrast, the myopathic features, such as weakness and muscle wasting, may persist despite maintenance of the euthyroid state."

Common Diseases and Syndromes of Body Pain

4.Neuromuscular status of thyroid diseases: a prospective clinical and electrodiagnostic study. (U.S. National Library of Medicine - PubMed) ---

Among the thyroid patients, 17 (42.5%) patients were diagnosed with mononeuropathy and polyneuropathy. Entrapment neuropathy was observed in 30% and diffuse neuropathy in 10% of the patients. Myopathy findings were observed in 2 patients.

5.Aspects of peripheral nerve involvement in patients with treated hypothyroidism. (U.S. National Library of Medicine - PubMed) ---

"RESULTS: Sixty-three per cent of the patients with 'pure' hypothyroidism had abnormalities on NCS, 25% had reduced IENF density and 31% had abnormalities on QST. Four patients (25%) met criteria for small fibre polyneuropathy, the other (75%) were classified as having mixed fiber polyneuropathy.

I believe this research makes the point very clear, that not all thyroid patients see recovery from neuropathy or myopathy symptoms, following proper treatment.

Co-morbid Nutritional Deficiencies

A final reason for treated thyroid patients continuing to experience neuropathy and/or myopathy symptoms or actually developing them in spite of being treated, that I will also mention, are "nutritional deficiencies" occurring co-morbid to thyroid disease.

All nutrients, which include vitamins, minerals and electrolytes, have potential to negatively affect nerve and/or muscle function when they become imbalanced and this can be true whether they become deficient or abnormally elevated in the body.

Common deficiencies that are found in thyroid patients include vitamins B12 and D and the mineral-electrolyte deficiencies potassium and magnesium. Others can potentially occur as well however, including deficiencies in other B-vitamins, as well as vitamin E and other types of essential nutrients.

When myopathy and/or neuropathy are occurring in spite of adequate thyroid treatment, a full nutritional blood panel should be ordered. All nutritional deficiencies are treatable and corrective supplementation of nutrients can correct problems in the nerves and muscles that are dependent upon normal levels of them.

Common Diseases and Syndromes of Body Pain

Hyperthyroid patients are at risk for developing nutritional deficiencies, due to their sped-up digestion, which causes food to pass through them very quickly. Most patients experience ongoing diarrhea and this can result in malabsorption of essential nutrients over time. Once their hyperthyroidism is corrected, they may still need low nutrients replaced via proper supplementation, as approved by their doctors.

My Own Diagnosis of Thyroid Disease and Deficient Nutrients

My case of Hashimoto's thyroiditis, diagnosed in year-2003 <u>has not</u> been passed down to me from previous generations. Neither my parents, grandparents nor even my great grandparents were known to have autoimmune thyroid disease of any kind. Some medical research, as stated by the AACE (American Association of Endocrinologist), states that thyroid autoimmunity is inherited in approximately 50% of cases that are diagnosed. In my case it is not inherited and my belief is that EBV (the "Epstein - Barr virus" -- that causes mononucleosis) is very possibly a direct cause of my autoimmune hypothyroidism. The correlations to contracting the virus in my childhood and to my ongoing immune system problems, from that point forward, are simply too striking to be coincidental.

When I was approximately age-10, I became very ill with mononucleosis and I was out of school with the virus for over 6 weeks. My two brothers and my sister never manifested any symptoms of mono, in spite of being in close contact with me during my bout with the illness. Once the viral illnesses had run its course, the glands in my neck returned to normal size, my fever resolved and my fatigue improved. I returned to school and normal activities but my body continued to manifest problems that I now know were related to dysfunction of my immune system. I developed childhood asthma and I experienced colds and viruses, more frequently than did my siblings. I remember on one occasion, my family contracted a respiratory virus and upon all of us our seeing a doctor on the same day, he informed my parents that my case was the most severe.

I mention this regarding EBV, due to the fact that many medical research studies have been published, linking EBV to the development of neurological conditions. This gives me yet one other possibility of a cause for both my thyroid autoimmunity and my co-morbid neuropathy symptoms.

My belief is that autoimmune thyroid diseases are among the common post-viral effects of EBV. I noticed some time ago, that an Oklahoma-based medical research group, was attempting to patent a vaccination for EBV.

Common Diseases and Syndromes of Body Pain

In their statements included on their patent application, they cite the fact that the virus has been implemented as a cause of many different autoimmune diseases. My feeling is that the immune system is adamant about eradicating the body of this virus. When it cannot do-so completely, it may begin to attack major organs or hormone glands that contain the virus, including a person's thyroid gland. This is a theory at this point but one I feel has real merit in light of medical research studies.

My Treatment since Year 2003

In my case as a hypothyroid patient, treated since 2003, with ongoing nerve and muscle symptoms, I was found to be deficient in vitamins D and E and I was found to have insufficient levels of B12 as well (low-normal).

My blood electrolyte level of potassium was found to be slightly below normal and my phosphate became slightly elevated, however, the phosphate normalized with replacing the low vitamin levels, while the potassium required supplementation and diet changes to correct.

Some thyroid patients can benefit from a good daily multivitamin and they can certainly benefit from modifying their diets to include more fruits, vegetables, nuts and grains.

117

This type of diet can help to combat the negative effects of neuropathy and/or myopathy, versus simple carbohydrates which come in the form of junk foods. Regular exercise helps nutrients and hormones to circulate better in the body and helps the body to rid itself of toxins and extra fat that can block some of the positive effects of nutrients.

CHAPTER FOUR

Considering all Treatment Options for Thyroid Neuropathy and Myopathy

Neuropathy and myopathy in thyroid disease patients can be improved in most cases to varied degrees as previously discussed. For some patients, these problems may completely resolve over time, while others may still experience them.

The first consideration in resolving these symptoms best-possible is to make sure thyroid hormone therapies are optimized, best possible. For some thyroid doctors, this means getting the TSH level suppressed into the low-normal or even the lowest-normal value and getting the T4 and T3 levels raised to above mid-range and possibly up to highest-normal values. Needs are varied among different patients and this is why it is important that a qualified doctor is sought for treatment and one who considers each patients' symptoms as well, rather than basing treatment on blood lab values alone.

Getting tested for possible nutritional deficiencies can also be very important as previously mentioned, especially if thyroid hormone correction does not adequately relieve muscle and nerve related symptoms.

CHAPTER FIVE

Eight Thyroid Disease Knock-Knock Jokes: (Laughing at the Expense of the Metabolic Butterfly)

Some readers might think "What! – A thyroid disease joke chapter – you've got to be kidding!" and I would respond by saying "Yes, I am kidding and that's the purpose of this chapter!" We're doing something that comedy often does, by taking a serious subject and finding a way to laugh about it. Why not?!

As thyroid patients who go through the ups and downs of our diseases, why shouldn't we find a way to derive some humor from it? I believe by doing so, that we can actually find better coping as we may sometimes struggle with the fact that we're living with a lifelong disease that will require ongoing treatment for most of us, as we live out our lives in this world.

What better way is there, to take some of the seriousness out of the fear we sometimes experience when we're having a flare of symptoms or we're experiencing some emotional phases with our diseases, than to find ways to laugh about it?

It is my sincere hope that fellow-patients or anyone who enjoys a good laugh will do-so, while reading this added bonus-chapter. As a patient with autoimmune thyroiditis that is causing me lifelong hypothyroidism and co morbid health problems, plus a need for daily treatments for it, I feel that laughter truly is a good medicine that can help me to cope better, when I'm feeling a bit down due to my disease and its symptoms. I hope this proves to be the case for those who read this chapter as well!

While some of these knock-knock jokes are a bit on the corny side (some smack in the middle of it), I think they will still get you to smile a little and hopefully some of them will get a few genuine giggles out of you. So, with the boring chapter-introduction out of the way, let's get to the comedy.

Knock-knock

Who's there?

I Goiter

I goiter who?

I goiter go to the doctor, cause my neck feels swollen.

Knock-knock

Who's there?

R.U. Goins

R.U. Goins who?

R.U. Goins to the doctor, cause your mood seems like it's hypothyroid.

_____

Knock-knock

Who's there?

I.M. Crabbie

I.M. Crabbie who?

I.M. crabbie because I forgot to take my thyroid pill this morning.

_____

Common Diseases and Syndromes of Body Pain

Knock-knock

Who's there?

B.A. Angel

B.A. Angel who?

B.A. angel and order me a double cheeseburger, my hypothyroidism is making me hungry.

Knock-knock

Who's there?

B4 U

B4 U Who?

B4 U call me a zombie, remember that I might be having brain fog.

Common Diseases and Syndromes of Body Pain

Knock-knock

Who's there?

I.R. Moody

I.R. Moody who?

I.R. Moody today, so don't push your luck by pushing my buttons.

Knock-knock

Who's there?

I.B. Shedding

I.B. Shedding who?

I.B. Shedding hair, so don't mistake my pillow for a raccoon in the bed.

Common Diseases and Syndromes of Body Pain

Knock-knock

Who's there?

M.I. Goen

M.I. Goen who?

M.I. goen to the doctor soon, cause my thyroid hormone pills don't seem to be working?

_____

About the Author:

I am a husband, father, grandfather and lifetime contract salesman, with experience in health writing that began in 2004. I completed theological studies with Liberty University in 1996. I formerly served as editor and forum moderator of Thyroid Health for a major multi-topic content site and as a general health writer for another, on which I achieved Editor's Choice Awards for my articles on health subjects.

In 2003 I was diagnosed with hypothyroidism; "Hashimoto's thyroiditis" being the cause. This autoimmune form of thyroid disease that causes destruction of the thyroid gland resulted in my also developing "Chronic Fatigue Syndrome", due to a compromised immune system with severe co-morbid "Adrenal Fatigue". I also suffered severe anxiety symptoms, including panic attacks early into the onset of Hashimoto's thyroiditis (Hashitoxicosis). I was also diagnosed with peripheral neuropathy and thyroid myopathy, with co-morbid nutritional deficiencies.

My eventual receiving of diagnoses was a difficult process with proper diagnostic testing not being ordered by the first doctors I sought treatment from.

Common Diseases and Syndromes of Body Pain

These types of issues were inspiration for me to become proactive in my own health care and to self-educate myself on these health disorders, which I have done extensively since 2003. I now enjoy sharing this information with other patients experiencing my same health disorders.

(END)